Praise for

FREE LOVE

World traveler Allie Chee's new book **Free Love** *is a delight to read with its bits of wisdom, common sense about healthy living, and feeling good about the simple things in life.*

— SCOTT E. MINERS

Editor, *Well Being Journal*

We are all on a quest for joy and happiness. We search, read, listen to "experts" for advice and still happiness eludes us.

In this simple book, Allie Chee shows us how to find utter joy in the simplest day-to-day things... things we take for granted or pass by or ignore as too simple.

Building true joy means embracing our experiences and using them to create the fabric of our daily lives. In **Free Love**, *Allie shows us how in her uniquely charming and honest way.*

— CHRISTINA PIRELLO

Emmy award-winning TV host of "Christina Cooks" and best-selling author

I love **Free Love.** *I love that it honestly explores how we make choices and dares to challenge the ones we are making collectively. I love that it is not preachy, yet inspires deep change in simple, practical ways. I love that it is written from the heart about living from the heart.*

Definitely a tool for helping us Be The Change that we wanna see. Buy your **Free Love** *now.*

— DR. CLAUDIA WELCH, DOM

Author, *Balance Your Hormones, Balance Your Life*

Thank you for sharing your wisdom at a time when American families need your advice most...

In **Free Love,** *the reader will find both a philosophical and prescriptive path to a new awareness of what truly matters.*

— JOY FELDMAN, NC, JD

Author, *Joyful Cooking in Pursuit of Good Health* and *Is Your Hair Made of Donuts?*

Bring on the free love! This book is a "being while doing" adventure guide through daily life in your own home. And you'll come back to it wanting your moment with Allie Chee and her tales of world travel that spice up every section, because her delightful personality imbues every page and makes you laugh again at the little stuff.

Don't get bogged down—get into free love!

— MICHELE RITTERMAN, PHD

Family Therapist, Author, *The Tao of a Woman*

While reading **Free Love**, *readers are taken on a path of awareness and self-discovery as they learn to embrace what truly matters to them in their everyday lives.*

Free Love *takes the notion of a simple everyday life and turns it into a daily journey of enlightenment and discovery. The ideas presented in the book are not complex, just easy changes of perspective that have a profound impact.*

— AMANDA SCHEWAGA

Co-founder, The Birthing Site

FREE LOVE

Other works by Allie Chee

NEW MOTHER

Using a Doula, Midwife, Postpartum Doula, Maid, Cook, or Nanny to Support Healing, Bonding and Growth

LOVE BATH

A Soak in Joy and Courage for Moms-to-be

(Scheduled for publication Spring 2013)

FREE LOVE

EVERYDAY IDEAS FOR JOYFUL LIVING

ALLIE CHEE

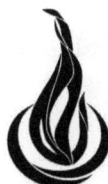

HESTIA
BOOKS & MEDIA

Published in the United States by
Hestia Books & Media
1111 West El Camino Real, #109-207
Sunnyvale, CA 94087

ISBN-13: 978-0-9856264-2-6

First Hestia Books & Media edition 2012.

Editorial team: David Colin Carr, Birgitte Rasine, Susan Monroe
Cover design by Laura Coyle
Interior illustrations by Jillian Dister
Interior layout by LUCITÀ Inc.

For more information about Allie Chee and her work, visit:
Web: www.alliechee.com
Blog: www.freelovebook.blogspot.com

Printed in the United States of America on FSC-certified, 30% post consumer recycled paper.

DEDICATION

In loving memory of Mother Teresa.

Thank you for taking the call from a lost soul in Laguna, looking to get her groove back.

And to YOU, Free Lover!

CONTENTS

Simple and easy ideas for the kitchen that anyone,
at any income level can implement—right now—to
instantly create:

- better health

- more quality family time

- and more love

ACKNOWLEDGMENTS

With Special Thanks To . . .

The people around the way who showed me free love. The list is long and spans the globe. Some are from my childhood, others I've known my whole life, others only moments.

Some of them are: Mrs. Silvia Jacobson, Sister Terry Ann, Tony Braubach, La Marquise de Brantes, Krystal and Heinrich Stumpf, Turkan Yukselen, Nicolai Sinkavich, Richard McGill, Julian Richard, Durga Dai, Dr. Henri Woo, Gary Beck, Rex and Reen Jaramillo, Kaku Singh and Maji, Papa Haj Ben Archour, Sharif Aberderahman, Irene Albert, Uli and Karl Heinz, Adrienne McMillan, Brother ChiSing Eng, Enriqueta Kleinman, Leo and Yshel Lok, Misha Steidl, and the citizens of Mostar, a people who—despite so much hardship and loss—shared with me otherworldly free love.

INTRODUCTION

My Hour with Mother Teresa

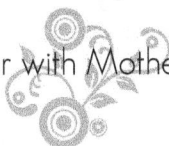

Let the beauty we love be what we do.
There are hundreds of ways to kneel and kiss the ground.

— *Rumi*

In 1993, I experienced something new and fantastic that I'd never known: freedom from fear about ability to pay the rent and the joy of being able to buy—within reason—any food, dwelling, car, clothing, jewelry, or vacation that I desired.

I'd been working since I was 13. I worked my way through college holding down two and even three jobs at a time. For the first time in about a decade, I had only one job (albeit a challenging one), no homework, and cash.

Party time!

Or so I thought.

I was living in Laguna Beach, I had a few good friends, and life *should* have felt pretty good. But when I read the top-selling book of the day, **Bridges of Madison County**, I burst out crying and didn't stop for about two days.

I remember lying on my futon, swollen eyes, throwing empty Kleenex boxes into a pile of tear-stained tissues strewn across the floor. The book struck a chord with a lot of people—it sold fifty million copies—and that was pre-Internet. But crying for two days and going through box after box of Kleenex? I knew I was dealing with something more than this book. Why? I was from Texas and I might shed a tear or two in private if someone passed on… but bawl like a baby over a little story?

For me, it was the story of a woman who'd accepted what was supposed to be "a good life," did what she believed was "right," but had not followed her heart's desire. The message to me was: You can have passion, travel, and excitement or the love and security of family—but not both. I don't know if I'd see it that way now—it's been 20 years since I read it—but that's the way I saw it then. I realized it struck a chord because not only was I not following my heart, I didn't even *know* where it wanted to go. Like so many people living as "transplants" in our country, I felt a serious lack of family, community, and love.

I started a journey of inner exploration, and over the following weeks I came to this conclusion:

I love Laguna, I enjoy making lots of money, and I love my friends. But I don't feel deep love or a sense of belonging in my life. Likely we all come to this conclusion at some point—or points—in our lives. When we do, we either hide in our work and busy-ness—or we start exploring, thinking, praying, trying to find meaning. This process is called *soul searching*. This was my time.

When we're in survival mode and busy beyond belief, we don't have time to dally with soul searching. Like being caught in the surf, we can't pause to enjoy the view of the horizon when trying to get through the next wave and maintain our breath. But once we break through the surf to calm, open water, we can pause for perspective.

It didn't take much soul searching for me to conclude that I'd made many decisions merely in the name of survival and financial gain and that my heart was lonely and longing. I was in love with work and travel. I wanted to see the world. I was also missing meaningful relationships. Maybe I had to accept that I couldn't have both. I decided that the only way to find true meaning and love was to set aside my personal passions and "give love away." But to whom?

My friends in Laguna had families and lifetime friends. Of course I could be a part of their lives, but those relationships couldn't go to the depths I wanted—at least not in a few months or even a few years. I wasn't in communication with my family, for healthy reasons, and wasn't about to look there. (Since that time, there's been a lot of healing and free love in the family!)

Lying on the beach one day, it hit me: *I'm going to Calcutta to work with Mother Teresa!*

(Random, but not as random as it might appear. I grew up in Catholic school and had even decided—in second grade—to be a nun when I grew up. I gave up that idea after praying under a tree, expecting the Virgin Mary to appear as she had in the movie they showed us in the convent at my school. She no-showed.)

That very evening I went home and called Mother Teresa. I called again and again. I don't know how many tries it took before I got a line through, but eventually I got to her. (India has come a long way in telecommunications since the early 90s.)

I spoke with her on the phone, as with an old friend, for about an hour. Only one hour with Mother Teresa changed the direction of my life forever.

She asked me why I wanted to come work with her, and I told her. This is what she told me:

"To learn to love is the most difficult and important thing we do."

"Your first job is to learn to love yourself. Many people fail to ever do this."

"Your next job is also very difficult, and only if you succeed in the first, and it is to learn to love your family."

"And then your next job, if and only if you succeed in the first two, is to learn to love your neighbors. Pick any neighbor, get to know them, care for them, and love them."

"And then, finally, if you've learned these three things— that would be a good time to identify strangers who could use your help. You said you live in the Los Angeles area? I imagine there are one or two needy people there. But if you still want to come work with me in India, there are always more people here who need help than those who are willing to, and you will be welcome."

Hmmm—what I needed was exactly what I had thought I needed—a lot of love in my life. And now I had an outline of how to go about giving, receiving, and living it.

Mother Teresa, a wise and loving mother.

She gave me many gifts in that call. She taught me that I didn't have to turn my back on the things I loved, the places I enjoyed, or the pursuit of financial gain to find my sense of belonging and true love in life. She taught me that I could find it anywhere I was or anywhere I wanted to be. And she set me on a path of learning to really give and receive love—which led around the world and back—several times. And to countless wonderful experiences I'd never dreamed of.

Traveling the world and finding so many people to love and learn from formed the basis of the ideas in this and all my works.

I hope that this book will serve as the "torch" that Mother Teresa gave me. I pass it along to you. At first glance, one might think: "Parties of One," cooking yams, dropping seeds into other people's pots, and walking barefoot—what's *that* got to do with learning to love ourselves and creating more meaning in life?

Wait and see. You *will* see.

PART 1:

HOW WE LOST OUR GROOVE

How We Lost Our Groove

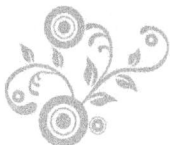

I n my book *New Mother: Using a Doula, Midwife, Postpartum Doula, Maid, Cook, or Nanny to Support Health, Bonding and Growth*, I discuss how profit-driven institutions have replaced the loving, natural experience of pregnancy and childbirth with cold, fear-driven template procedures.

Women and our entire society have conceded to a compromised experience out of fear and ignorance. But then at least three generations of women in the United States have grown up with this limited and mechanical vision of motherhood.

It doesn't have to be that way. In *New Mother*, I offer a delightful vision and specific instructions for reclaiming the natural, healthy, and sacred experience of motherhood.

In *Free Love*, we'll consider how the same profit-driven institutions have destroyed simple, healthy family lifestyles and structures—"villages"—with factory foods, TVs, and vacuous materialism... and what we can do about it.

And just what can little-ol' we do?

Move mountains!

We don't need to wait for the next election and hope to create change from a political perspective. We don't have to petition the corporations and hope that they will work for their customers' best interests.

We can make immediate, instant changes—all on our own—that will change the direction of our families' lives forever and benefit generations to come. As I learned from Mother Teresa, we don't have to give up anything that really gives us joy in the process.

There are ways we can reclaim the responsibilities and joy of caring for our home and families—even if we work fulltime, even on limited incomes. Listen up, friends!

I grew up in Texas in the 1960s and '70s. That was a unique time in world history. For the first time, women had completely conceded the care of their pregnancies and families to institutions. Gone was the network of family members and neighbors who genuinely cared for one another, who would share evenings together on the porch swapping stories. Gone were the women who stayed at home watching the children and cooking real food from scratch. The men were already out of the home, so with the women and extended families gone… no one was left.

Where did they go?

To work in jobs.

And what happened when they did?

The U.S. government says:

Stress and tension between work and family are increasing. Major changes in American families—and the lack of corresponding changes in many workplace policies and practices—are the causes. [1]

---

1. United States Department of Labor, Office of the Secretary on the Internet, http://www.dol.gov (April 2012).

And I say:

"Stress and tension" indeed! We've lost our groove!

Specifically:

Many of us here in the U.S. rarely cook.

Not only do we not cook, we don't know *how* to cook, and haven't for at least three generations. I'm generalizing—there are exceptions—please bear with me. I'm working on the premise that opening boxes, cans, and microwaving is not cooking.

We leave not just our older children, but also *newborns* sometimes only a few weeks old, to the care of strangers.

New mothers often have a maximum of six weeks—that's 42 days—to spend raising their infants before they turn them over to daycare or a nanny. If mom decides to take a few of those weeks as "vacation" before her baby arrives, then her postpartum leave is even less. In any branch of medicine, the newborn isn't even considered fully developed until three months old—but they're being yanked from their parents' care at six tiny weeks.

We allow pharmaceutical companies and food conglomerates to feed our babies.

"Though first developed by Henri Nestlé in the 1860s, infant formula received a huge boost during the post-World War II Baby Boom." [2]

According to a National Immunization Survey (NIS) under the direction of the CDC,[3] nationwide in 2010, of the infants who were then 19-35 months of age:

• 75% were breastfed at birth; that dropped to 43% by six months, and only 13% of those were exclusively breastfed

• Only 33% were exclusively breastfed at three months

Of course, there are some cases in which the mother has trouble nursing or the baby has trouble latching, but let's ask why so many are having trouble. If we ask—rather than immediately offering formula samples—we probably won't need to look far to find reasons.

---

2. "Baby Boomer," Wikipedia, The Free Encyclopedia, http://en.wikipedia.org/wiki/Baby_Boomer (April 2012).
3. "Breastfeeding Benefits & Barriers: Breastfeeding Statistics in the United States," http://www.breastfeedingbasics.org/cgi-bin/deliver.cgi/content/Introduction/sta_us.html (April 20, 2012).

Too often, grandparents and extended family aren't involved and don't support new moms.

Once highly depended upon for childcare, cooking, wisdom, homemaking skills, and love they could impart, grandparents have little or no role or value in the family beyond a friend who visits, in some cases often but in many cases, rarely. Extended family members all live in separate homes and cities, each struggling to maintain their own nuclear families.

This, of course, leaves a great percentage of the elderly alone and inactive, in front of TV screens day in and day out, and tucked safely away in "retirement communities" until they finally expire. *No love!*

Family health—physical and mental—is suffering.

- Too many parents (fortunately not all) are overworked and exhausted while serving the two masters of career and family.

- Stress and disease due to poor diet affect almost every home (Considering pharmaceutical sales, divorce, obesity, and alcoholism statistics, it may be that *every* home is affected in one way or another.)

- An ever-growing percentage of children are sick, overweight, sedated (given legal and taking illegal drugs), and neglected. So much so that it's considered *normal* for children to be frequently sick and taking medication regularly. It isn't normal for infants to throw up all the time; for children to bounce off the walls in a dizzy haze or anger; or for them to have the new respiratory infection, digestive tract dysfunction, or rash of the week. Common—yes. Natural—no.

• The most common form of entertainment for the individual or family group is staring at a screen, which is very likely flashing highly violent and hateful images or scenes (sometimes clipped so quickly that our brains are not designed to process them).

Our neighborhoods have been reduced to rows of dwellings with a strip mall somewhere in the vicinity.

Neighborhoods have little sense of friendship and community. Big neighborhood bookstore chains have pushed out the little neighborhood bookstores, and chain cafes have pushed out the mom-and-pops. Now even the "big ones" are bankrupt and closing. Where is the community center or meeting place?

What's going on? How did all this happen?

These are the results of *losing a war.*

World War II Ends and World War III Begins

In the early1800s, families worked almost exclusively on their own farms and were essentially self-sufficient. By 1850, men were leaving the farms to find work in factories. By 1900, almost 19% of women over 16 were finding work outside the home, but less than 6% of married women worked outside the home.[4]

Until the 1920s, the role of the married woman in the home was clear, solid, and respected. She either ran the household by managing servants (the minority), or she ran her home as women had for millennia—through hard work, dedication, and service to her family by caring for children, cooking, and cleaning.

The Great Depression in the 1930's, followed by World War II, changed all that.

During the Depression, women were encouraged—and many had no choice—to leave the home and enter the workplace. During WWII, again they were encouraged to take up jobs in factories and plants left by men in the service. And that they did.

Between 1940 and 1945, the female percentage of the U.S. workforce increased from 27% to nearly 37%.[5]

---

4. "Women in the Labor Force," http://www.infoplease.com/ipa/A0104673.html (April 20, 2012).
5. "American Women in World War II," History.com, http://www.mscd.edu/history/camphale/www_001.html (August 24, 2012).

Another thing happened as women entered the workforce in the 1940s that deeply affected the family: the television. In 1946, 8,000 U.S. homes had TV. Only 10 years later that number was 35 million. By 1970, 96% of American homes had a television in *at least* one room.[6] Now, take a look at these statistics:

- Number of minutes per week that parents spend in meaningful conversation with their children: 3.5

- Number of minutes per week that the average child watches television: 1,680

- Hours per year the average American youth watches television: 1500

- Hours per year the average American youth spends in school: 900[7]

The high priests of behavioral psychology refined their art, and they have had progressively greater reach selling beliefs fabricated for commercial gain through print, radio, Internet, and TV.

---

6. "Baby Boomers in Hot and Cold Wars," Farming in the 1950s and 60s, http://www.livinghistoryfarm.org/farminginthe50s/life_01.html (April 2012).
7. "Television & Health," Internet Resources to Accompany the Sourcebook for Teaching Science, http://www.csun.edu/science/health/docs/tv&health.html (April 2012).

Take both parents out of the home and bring the TV in to "occupy" the infants and children, and World War III begins in America—the war on the family. With no one to protect the fort (home) and a secret agent (the screen) having infiltrated almost every room of every house, there has been a steady and ever-increasing onslaught of chemical weapons released on the family: factory food, plastic and toxic cooking tools and methods, chemical cleaning agents, plastic (synthetic) clothing, an avalanche of pharmaceuticals, and more.

For the majority of the middle class (not the lowest income strata)—in other words, for most Americans—both parents are needed in the workforce fulltime *only* to support excess consumption. Some examples:

- Two relatively new cars (less than 5-7 years old)

- The current American "style" of family life requires three to five times more physical space than anywhere else in the world—meaning homes sufficient in size that family members can effectively avoid each other and that can rack up $300, $500, even $1,000 air conditioning bills in summer.

- Clothing and accessories in extraordinary excess of what is necessary—for example, frames for glasses and sunglasses that cost $100-$500 each

- $60 mani-pedis and $350 foil highlights

- Parents' hobbies: golf, tennis, drinking

- Designer children's clothing—piles of it

- Hundreds of junky toys for children that wind up stuffed in garages or in landfills

- Private gym memberships

- Accessories, "fancy" food, and boarding for pets

- The ironic daycare and restaurant expenses necessary since so many people aren't home

- Many people work two jobs and incur a lifetime of debt so they can buy a house in the "right" school district, incidentally incurring a lifetime of stress and compromised family time.

I know people who are living with what is considered the very lowest income who still indulge in many of these luxuries.

Who am I to be saying this? And just what am I gettin' at?

Let's clear the air before I have people on all sides riled up.

- I don't—as I know most other women don't—want to give up our hard-earned freedoms in the name of family…and I don't think we have to (the point of this book)!

- It doesn't have to be "just the women" raising and caring for the family. Hopefully it's not. Details coming up!

- Sometimes people confuse discussions about the negative effects of excessive materialism with communist tendencies. All I can say to that is a big, resounding, "Nyet!" I witnessed the results of communist oppression in 10 countries that are currently working to climb their way into material wealth and some sense of spirituality and ethics. Hopefully that plague has had its run.

- No ascetic tendencies in me, either. The "greed is good" philosophy is nonsense. Greed is always ugly. But the desire to climb ever higher in creativity and all forms of abundance—that's the definition of nature itself. That desire serves to motivate and encourage learning and personal growth. I enjoy thoroughly living in material abundance— *just not if it's at the expense of my family,* meaning our time together or our health.

And that's the point. Many families claim they can't afford to live on one or reduced income. Yet, they often can. However, if we choose "things" in excess over family, it's time to recognize that **we're not poor. We've simply made a poor choice.**

I say these things with sympathy and understanding for those in the struggle (whether self-induced by overconsumption or legitimate). I've experienced a wide range of financial existence.

On the low side: At age 13 I worked at Haagen-Dazs® scooping ice cream so I could buy the "little extras," like food and basic toiletries. I've spent plenty of time looking at bare cupboards and wondering whether paying the rent or buying groceries was going to make the budget cut for the week. I had to drop out of college when I broke my leg one summer. Losing my ability to work for three months cost me the income I needed to pay for tuition, books, and rent. I cried and cried when they put that cast on my leg—not because it hurt, but because I wondered if, along with college, I'd also lose my car.

On the other side, I've been what I considered well off. I've never been afraid of work and have been happy to hold down three jobs at a time to get out of a month-to-month existence. That tenacity and desire, after decades of application, paid off.

Before getting married—and almost 20 years out of college—I had a 3,200 square foot house with a pool (with only little ol' me living there), a convertible Mercedes (CPO, paid cash), and I spent plenty of dough on the offerings in piazzas and duty-frees around the world. If I saw a necklace I wanted, I called it "art." One doesn't question the price of fine art. If I saw a $3,000 leather coat in the Versace window in Verona, I'd call it "a priceless memory of my travels," and I'd wear it on the plane home. $200 for the smoked salmon "lunch pack" at my favorite boutique in Heathrow... well, airplane food is inedible, so of course I'll take two to hold me over on my long flight wherever.

My work over the years had provided a fairly handsome income—which likely would have continued.

However, when we got married, my husband and I decided to adjust our lifestyle so that *no matter what*, we could live without depending on two incomes and I could stay at home full-time with our children. We didn't need to give up *all* the extras, but to be safe and assure the home life we wanted, we cut back in a lot of areas. If we'd married and had children younger in life, we surely would have had to make deeper cuts in the material standard of living—which neither of us would hesitate to do now if it were necessary.

Though our society has come a long way from such conditions—fortunately—we don't need more than a one-room dwelling; one set of clothing and a coat, unless the climate is warm (and then we wouldn't need any clothing); and if we had none and really wanted jewelry, we could string some shells together, add a few pretty rocks, and—*hey*—isn't that what designers charge thousands for?

I've schlepped up muddy, washed-out roads to visit people in shantytowns of cardboard-box dwellings in the hills of Mexico.[8] In a gas station (more accurately, gas shack) on the way there, I asked the attendant if I could use the restroom. He was very kind and polite but said emphatically, "No! Es muy sucio!" I'd used dozens of strange and horrible facilities around the world, so I insisted. After only seconds in the bathroom, I ran for fresh air, gagging, with tears streaming from my eyes, preferring the wide open road.

But I encountered a culture that can, even when extremely poor, put on a family fiesta with 50 people that goes on for days—for a baby's birthday.

---

8. These were not religious missions. I've traveled in approximately 50 countries, visiting each one for a different reason, but the overriding reason for all my travels has been fascination. I note this because many of the visitors to these places whom I met were doing charitable work—working to convert people. I wasn't there to teach. I was there to learn.

I've traveled two days by boat down a jungle river in the Miskito Coast of Honduras to villages with no electricity or water, staying with people living in a one-room hut on stilts and eating a diet of beans and rice for breakfast, beans and rice for lunch, and for dinner... you guessed it. Fruit, vegetables, and meat were extraordinary indulgences and hard to come by. While I was there, two ten-year-olds were sent on a two-day trip down the river to trade an entire canoe of bananas for a pound of coffee beans with another village. The most educational experience I had there was seeing three-year-old girls wearing slings on their backs bearing their infant siblings. It was their job to watch the infants while mothers tended the fields.

But most important, I saw a community that supported each other in every aspect of life—from field, to flock, to food, to fun.

I've been in the back alleys of China and seen whole families living in single rooms with a bare bulb hanging from the 300-year old ceiling and a single sink that served all "water" needs. China has experienced tremendous growth and increase in wealth... but not *all* of China.

However, I saw an ancient code of respect and courtesy in place in even the most "lowly" of neighborhoods.

In 1990, I stayed with Russians (highly educated people able to converse on any topic of history, politics, and art), living three families to an apartment—one family in each of the two bedrooms and one family in the living room. In the one bathroom they all shared, I called out for my friend Nicholai to pass me some toilet paper (having found none next to the toilet). He called back, "Newspaper on floor not for reading."

In Moscow with my friend Nastya, we were driven around town by her boyfriend Maxim. (He was extremely wealthy to have a car—a Lada—at the young age of 22.)

He arrived a bit late, said something to Nastya in Russian, and then she screamed, "You didn't get gas yet!" Wanting to restore the peace without understanding the situation, I chimed in, "Hey, let's just get gas on the way." Maxim smiled and she groaned—and soon I knew why.

We turned off a main street and screeched to a halt behind a snarled, tangled mess 15 cars wide and perhaps a block long. I could see the gas station in the distance. In the immediate scene were people, with their car engines turned off, sitting on the hoods and trunks playing cards, drinking, or staring into space. *Three hours later*, we had gas and were off to sightsee. I'd already seen the most important sight of the day.

Most striking against this backdrop of corruption and poverty in Russia was the incredible emphasis on education. People waiting in line four hours for milk (me, with them) could speak three or four languages with perfect fluency.

In 2001, I traveled though Lebanon and saw a gorgeous country with more than half its buildings and neighborhoods still shattered from a 17-year civil war that had ended 11 years earlier.

BUT, oh, is Beirut fun in the summer! Food, family, and music dominate the day.

That same year I drove to Bratislava, Slovakia—a charming and fascinating town. I stood on a hilltop on the grounds of what was a medieval fortress and saw the telltale sign of Soviet rule below in the city: rows and rows of hideous cinder block, vodka- and urine-soaked buildings called "housing." From up on the hill, they looked like tombstones. I've spent the better part of a year living in that kind of building in Soviet-run countries, and they felt like graveyards.

Yet, the café life in Bratislava rivals any small town in Europe: block after block of charming restaurants and cafes, sidewalks lined with tables and bright umbrellas, people enjoying their town *al fresco*!

In 2003, I drove through Bosnia and Herzegovina. Fresh out of a vicious war that resulted in the breakup of Yugoslavia, I saw the result of great destruction and hatred. In one of the border towns (I don't know the names of any small cities I drove through—all the signs were in Cyrillic) was the embodiment of devastation. There wasn't one person to be seen, yet thousands—yes, thousands—of graves were scattered around any empty field. Even the tombstones were bullet-riddled. I walked through the crushed remains of people's homes. Most haunting was standing in what had been someone's kitchen, finding weeds growing over shards of lovely, but crushed, dishware. Everywhere, car chassis like rotting skeletons were turned over, burned-out, shot-up, and rusted.

Despite the enormity and recent occurrence of the violence there, I was blown away when I saw downtown Sarajevo. While the civil war had largely been of a religious nature, I saw thousands of U.N. police carrying machine guns—yet—I saw people: old and young, wearing hijabs and kippahs, traditionally dressed and scantily dressed, all strolling and sitting together in what looked like a bustling, happy life. I was enchanted and literally cried tears of joy.

When people say, "You need to face reality," I laugh and wonder *which one?* Reality is always in the eye of the beholder, and even then, multi-faceted and elusive.

But still, the term "reality check" comes to mind when friends in the U.S. say things to me along the lines of, "You simply CANNOT have a baby without owning an SUV." Or when digging through a mountain of clothing in the child's room, "I can't find anything for him to wear!" Or, "It's their future... your toddler must have a cell phone and tablet." The worst part is, it's not hyperbole—they believe it.

You see the point—I've experienced the wealth and the struggle in poverty, as well as the poverty and blessings in wealth. And here in the U.S., even if we cut way, Way, WAY back to accommodate our shifting desires to spend more time with family, the majority of us still have it very good and indeed have the ability to achieve our goals.

I know a handful of couples that have made the choice that my husband and I did for their families—and two of them are my cousins. Interestingly, they both married women who had extremely successful careers, and both women decided that raising their children and cooking three meals a day for their families meant more to them than the extra luxuries and security that two incomes could provide. (I discuss this from my view of a woman staying home with children, since women are the ones best equipped to feed and care for the infant—initially. Of course, fathers can be the ones to work less away from home, or not at all, to care for the family.)

I'm sure there are millions of couples that have made similar decisions—but they are likely not the majority. The statistics on the general condition of families, their health, eating habits, activities, and education all support that conclusion.

WHAT CAN WE DO?

Parents are exhausted by trying to serve the two masters of family and career. No servant can serve two masters—both masters receive compromised versions of the service they deserve, and the servant is run into the ground. After leaving their jobs away from home, parents race home to rapid-fire prepare something called food and relentlessly drive their children around town for activities with people who are little better than strangers.

Why do they do this? I'd guess if you asked them, they'd say, "For my kids." And I'm sure they mean it. Many believe they are providing better education for their kids and better job prospects (more money, ability to stay employed, etc.). It's what their parents did for them and what their grandparents did for their parents.[9]

In other words, they don't know any other way. How could they? Where are the examples? Where are the models of one parent as primary homemaker and one parent as primary financial provider honored in the U.S.? Where are family, friends, and community held in higher regard than "more stuff?"

At least one place—right here in this book!

I—and I believe thousands, if not millions, of other Americans—have started...

---

9. The "soccer mom" racing furiously around town for activities is a relatively new phenomenon, but the working mom, latchkey kid, and faux food experience have been going on for at least three generations.

- Asking *why?* Why would I race to work and then turn around and give a ton of money to daycare, restaurants, and food factories?

- Asking *what if?* What if we cut back here and there and one of us stayed home—even part-time—to care for our children, at least the first few or even five years of their lives?

- Asking *how?* I want to be with my kids, for our family to be healthy, for us to have more fun and peace in our lives... but how?

- Single people are asking, *what about life alone?* Can I find more love and joy in my life by myself?

- Single parents are asking the hardest question of all: *How?* How can I care for my kids better and create more peace and joy in our home when I must work such long hours?

- Finally, some people may be thinking, "What you say is all fine and good, Allie. I'd like a healthier, more loving family life and community, but *we're not changing our jobs or home structure.*"

No matter what you're asking or thinking, I've got some seriously fun, healthy, loving ideas for you to start using in your life this very minute.

I don't have all the answers, but for those looking, I have the answer for reclaiming our health, happy home life, and thriving community—right now, at any income level, and with even the smallest amount of free time.

PHOTO GALLERY

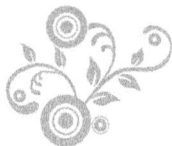

A t any time, no matter what the conditions, where there are
two or more people, there can be free love.

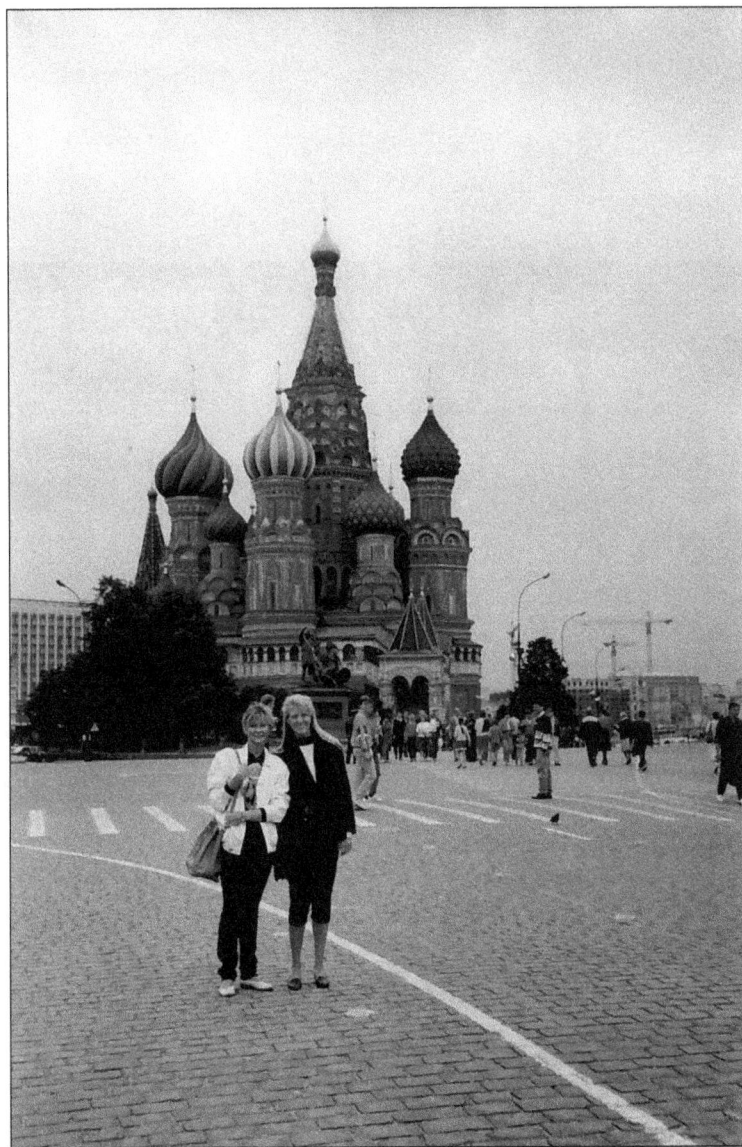

Photo courtesy of Allie Chee

**With a hard-won full tank of gas, we made it to Red Square
Russia, 1990**

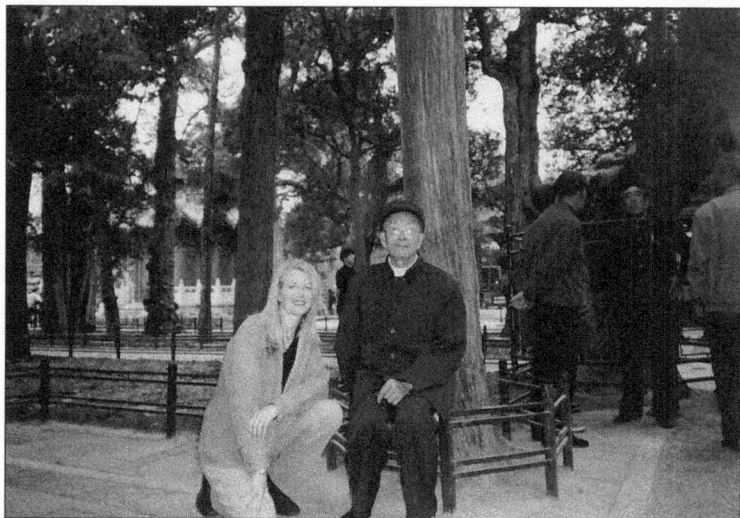

An image of a world quickly disappearing
Hangzhou, 2000

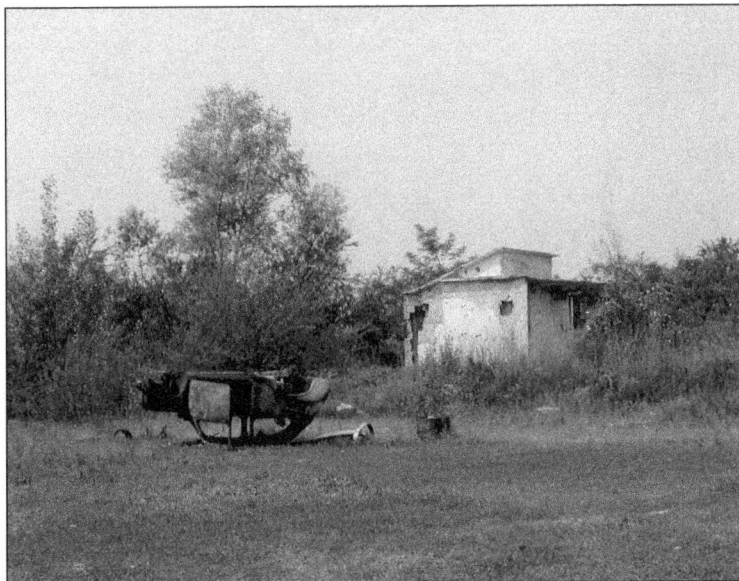

Photo courtesy of Allie Chee

Ghost town in Bosnia and Herzegovina, 2003

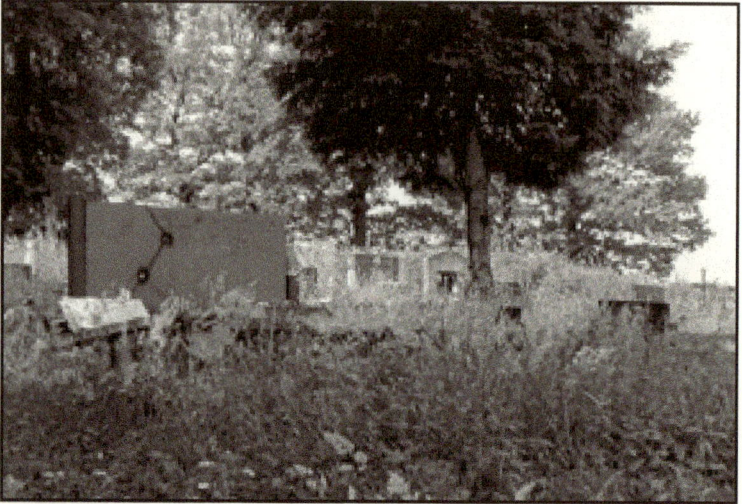

The ubiquitous view of gravestones
Bosnia and Herzegovina, 2003

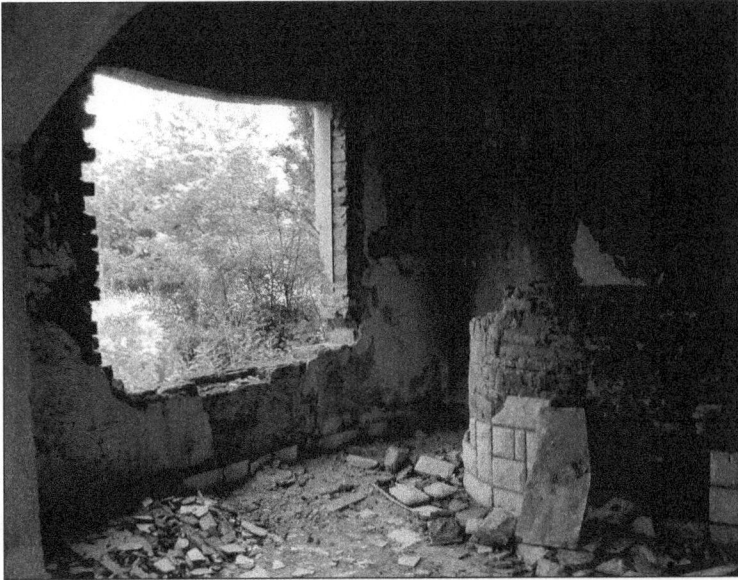

Photo courtesy of Allie Chee

The remains of a kitchen
Bosnia and Herzegovina, 2003

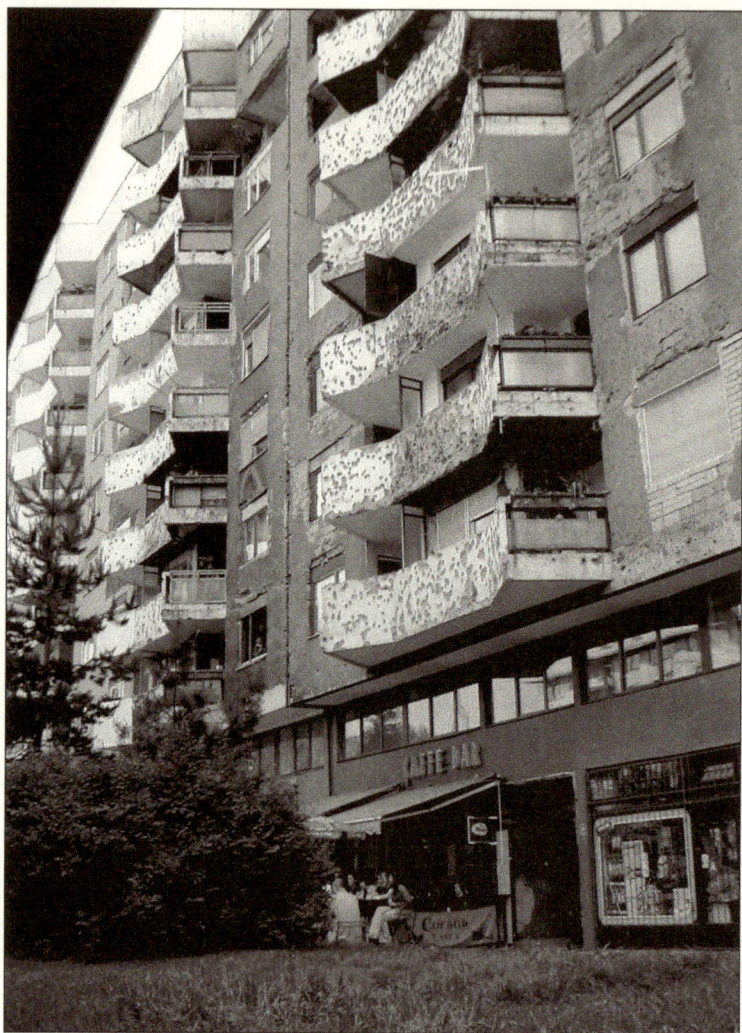

Photo courtesy of Allie Chee

***In a bullet-riddled building, a bustling cafe
and return to free love
Bosnia and Herzegovina, 2003***

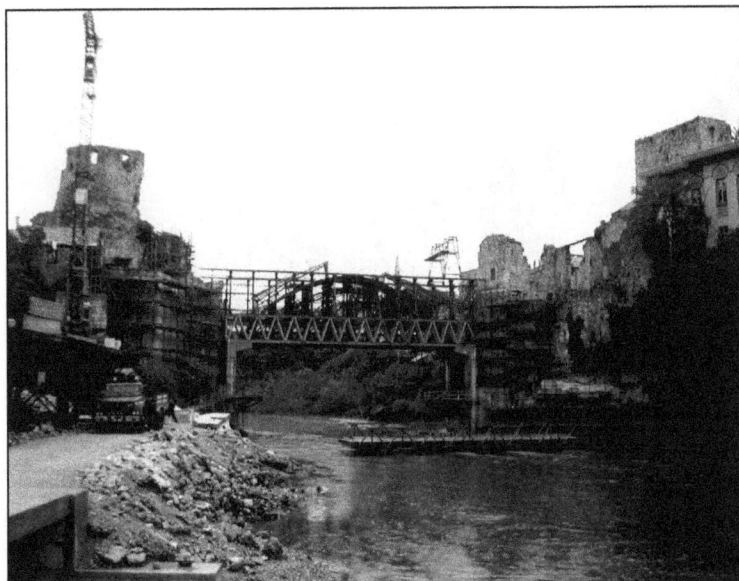

Photo courtesy of Allie Chee

The Mostar Bridge under reconstruction:
an international symbol of free love
Mostar, 2003

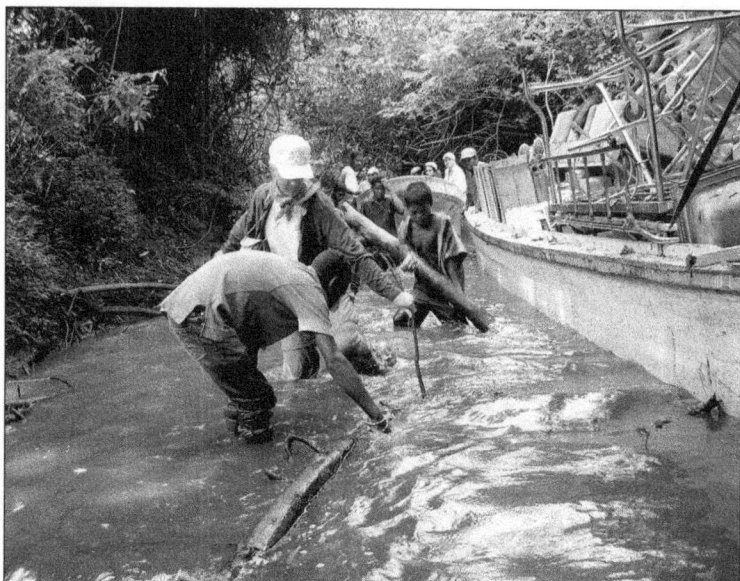

Photo courtesy of Allie Chee

Slow going down river
Miskito Coast, Honduras, 2005

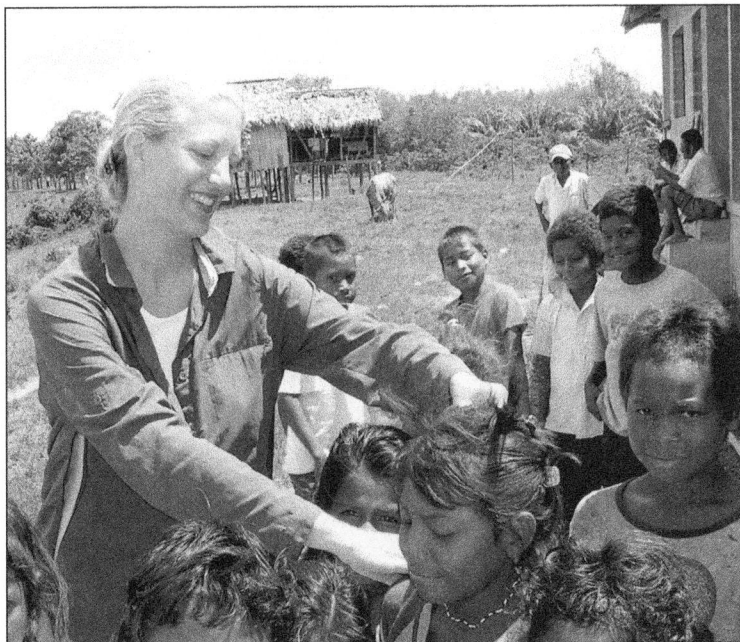

Photo courtesy of Allie Chee

**Village on the Coco River near the
Honduras-Nicaragua border, 2005**

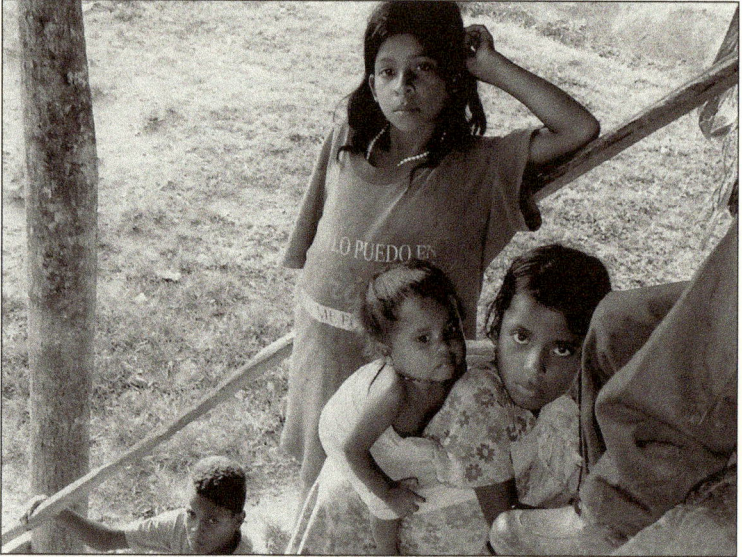

Girls 3-5 years old care for infant siblings
while mothers work the fields
Honduras, 2005

PART 2:

HOW WE GET OUR GROOVE BACK

A poor man celebrates the new year once a year.
A rich man celebrates each day.
But the richest man celebrates every moment.

– SRI SRI RAVI SHANKAR

AT THE HEARTH

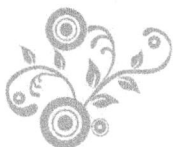

S imple and easy ideas for the kitchen that anyone, at any income level, can implement—right now—to instantly create:

- *Better health*

- *More quality family time*

- *And more love*

I use "hearth" to refer to the physical place in our house where we prepare our food—the kitchen, the stove, the literal fire—but also spiritually to refer to the "fire center" of the home where we create energy for the family. More energy = more love!

It's time for us to return to the hearth, to return to our role as creators of energy for the family. We've conceded this sacred space to factories, machines, and corporations, reducing the hearth to a microwave display space and factory food pantry.

We know all the reasons why we have allowed this: too little time, too little money, too little knowledge, and too little desire… and… we bought "the story" that our lives would be better this way. The story sounded good—but it's had its run and proven otherwise.

All that changes right here, right now.

You don't need a lot of money. You don't need a lot of time. You don't need a lot of knowledge.

The only thing you need is to search your feelings, follow your intuition, and remember this sacred truth: You are responsible for your health and your family's—now and for the next seven generations. If you're reading this, you're likely ready to reclaim your place at the family hearth and to own your position as matriarch or patriarch.

The following ideas are so simple that you can implement them right now when you take a break from reading.

No concern or excuse can stand in your way.

"I don't know how to cook."

Yes, you do, just perhaps not very well right now. That doesn't matter in the least. These are all simple ideas.

"I don't have the money to buy quality food."

Yes, you do. If organic or exotic foods are out of the budget now, you don't need them. Start where you are. There are countless foods you can afford—that will prove less expensive than factory foods—and that will bring more vitality to your family.

"I don't have time."

Yes, you do. Again, start where you are. If you don't have time to prepare feasts, or even three simple meals a day, start by cooking one meal a day… or even one meal a week.

We'll take this hill one step at a time and discover just how high you can climb in the next pages of this book and years of your life!

"I don't like to cook."

We can learn to love to cook. I'll share ideas of how I went from a diet of frozen and fast food to loving cooking three organic meals from scratch—every day—for my family. I've grown to consider it one of the greatest expressions of love for my family and myself.

The Italians have a saying: *Piano, piano!* It was the very first expression I learned when I lived in Italy because I heard it so often, and because the Italians are experts at *piano, piano!* It means "slowly, slowly" and implies that there's no worry, no need to rush—all things in good time.

That will be our mantra for every idea in this book. No need to feel overwhelmed. You can learn anything, you can learn to love anything, you can do whatever you want, you can change your life and claim health and beauty for generations to come—but—*piano, piano!*

So that's enough *piano, piano!* for now—let's get going!

If, after that assurance and encouragement, you still dread the thought of going into the kitchen and trying something new, just skip it for now and go immediately to the next section: "Free Love at Home."

If you're in a "dread mindset," it's not the time to try. But if you start implementing the great ideas in "Free Love at Home" and "Free Love Around the Way," you may find that soon your dread has transmuted into curiosity and enthusiasm regarding the kitchen.

Party of One

I was fresh out of a long relationship and stinging. You've felt that before. Not like an ant-bite sting. The sting where you can't sleep, can't eat, and wonder which way is up, and wonder how you'll go on. I decided the best thing to do would be: Go to the gym? Go to a bar? Stay home and feel wretched?

I decided the best thing to do was to fly to Buenos Aires and tango for two weeks!

That trip was exactly what the doctor ordered. I sat in the famous La Biela sipping cappuccino (that was right before I stopped drinking coffee) during the day and pouring my heart out in my journal. I strolled the incredible bookstores of Buenos Aires. I spent my evenings watching the best of the best dancers in the world's best *milongas*. I found one of the top teachers there and had a few private dance lessons.

I almost forgot that I'd been feeling horrible and why I'd flown there, until...

"Sola?" *Only one?* The *maître d'* asked me at the restaurant.

Ugh!

"Not only one!" I wanted to scream. "Party of one! Can't you see I'm not alone? I'm in the great company of a *milonguera* and having fun! I'm with myself!"

"Si, sola," I moaned, and he lead me to the pitiful, small table in the back next to the kitchen door that was for the "solos and solas." I pulled out my journal and wrote a string of scathing insults to that poor man.

If we are *sola*, we can find love in that. As Mother Teresa said, that's our first job. For me, one of the first steps in finding that self-love was to cook for myself. Full meals. Beautiful, healthy meals.

Most readers will be thinking what I used to think: *But it's such a drag to cook for just myself.*

Treat yourself as you would treat a baby, your best friend, or your lover. Cook gorgeous food for yourself and put flowers on the table! Put on great music and eat by candlelight! See if you don't fall in love!

(But, "I don't know how to cook," or "It takes too long," you say. Keep reading. By the time you put down this book, you won't be saying that.)

Inversely, if you aren't solo, invite your solo friends for meals *often!* Even though I encourage people to love cooking and caring for themselves, after too long and too many meals alone… it can start to feel like *just one*. If we know there are neighbors, family members, colleagues, or friends who live by themselves, invite them over to dine with you and your family as often as you can— don't wait for Thanksgiving or Christmas.

Have "Parties of five" all the time. Who doesn't love a party?

We celebrate everything.
Celebration is our way to receive all the gifts from God.

— Osho

Git it Gone!

I knew a woman in Texas who was big into the plastic surgery movement, and when I say *big*, y'all know what I'm sayin'.

Not only did she use plastic surgery to make additions, but she also used it to eliminate anything that could offend: wrinkles, smile lines, moles, hair, and fat. If she saw anything she didn't like in the mirror, she'd holler, "Git it gone!" and off she'd go to the surgeon.

I love that mantra. I can be heard shouting it in my kitchen, too. But I use it for things I don't want in, on, or around my body, not my body itself.

The very simplest, fastest, and FREE way to start improving our health is to eliminate the most offensive or destructive things we do.

Rather than a life overhaul—which, most often, doesn't work for a minute—I like to approach any project like this (one that may seem daunting at first glance) with a "Rule of 3." My

Rule of 3 is: Pick the three things from the list that are the very easiest for me to do, not do, or whatever required.

For cooking, we'll be looking at picking three things from a list of "food" items that we can stop eating immediately—things that we really won't miss and that are negatively affecting our health. After we adjust to living without those offenses—a day, a week, or six months from now—we pick three more to eliminate, and so on.

Below is a list of things I eliminated or changed over the course of 20 years. I won't include all the science, study, and research I found that led me to believe that these were offensive to health. You can conduct a study of nutrition if you're interested, use common sense, or just take my word for it. Look over my list or write your own. Then pick the three items you'll eliminate today and *Git it gone!*

Allie's *Git it Gone* list:

- Nonsense beverages: Includes "energy" drinks, sodas, and faux juices

- Food coloring and flavor enhancers

- Artificial sweeteners—all of them

- Anything with hydrogenated oils

- Artificial spreads, such as margarine

- Processed cheeses or anything that "squirts" out of plastic and makes sounds that are more appropriate for the restroom than the kitchen. *Git it gone!*

- Yogurt processed into a dessert with fillers, flavors, etc.—especially if it's marketed to children. You can count on those products to be compromised nutrition.

- Ice cream, any flavor, any brand, organic or not

- All chips and most crackers (basic principle: anything with more than four ingredients)

- Frozen, pre-prepared foods. Frozen peas: OK. Frozen pizza: *Git it gone!*

- Low-fat anything. If you want to lose weight, eat better foods—not equal amounts or more of "low-fat" processed foods.

- Store-bought desserts. If you home-make oatmeal cookies with oats, wheat flour, eggs, brown sugar, butter, and vanilla... it's not necessarily "health food," but it's great compared to store-bought, brand-name desserts, and "treats."

- Processed breakfast cereals. If you like cereal in the morning, the coming pages will tell you how to make delicious, nutritious, and inexpensive breakfast porridge from whole grains.

- Canned soup. In the coming pages, you'll find ideas for easily making incredibly delicious soups—without the added chemicals and salt. Try just one of those store-bought soups minus the salt, flavorings, and flavor enhancers (namely MSG and autolyzed yeast extract), and you'll never take a bite again.

- Any processed meats. Animals—just plain cuts of muscle, organ, or bone come with enough problems and reasons to consider changes in our diet. But processed meats come with all those problems, plus a lot more.

- For the grand finale: It's not a food item. It's the microwave. If you can't get rid of it (because it belongs to your landlord or would leave a gaping hole above your stove), use it as I do—unplug it and use it as a storage space for all your herbal teas.

There is absolutely nothing beneficial to health that needs to go in the microwave. If you need to thaw something, place it in a bowl of warm water, or leave it on the counter for a few hours or in the fridge for a day or two. If you need to reheat something, it's almost as fast in a saucepan or a toaster oven. And if you need to cook something—use the stove, oven, crock-pot, or grill.

There is a lot of research available about the negative effects of using a microwave, but how about we just ask a simple question:

Why are we warned to stand away from a microwave while it's in operation and how is it "detrimental" if we don't? [10]

I don't need to wait for the answer, and neither do you.

Aside from health benefits, everything will taste better. Once you're no longer accustomed to it, even the texture of food from a microwave will seem nasty.

I trust some of you must be shaking your heads, thinking: "If I got rid of all those things, the kitchen would be empty!"

---

10. "Commercial Microwave Oven Safety," http://www.foodservicewarehouse. com/restaurant-equipment-supply-marketing-articles/product-safety-public-health/commercial-microwave-oven-safety/c28214.aspx (August 24, 2012).

I know, because that's exactly what I thought when I read ideas like this twenty years ago. I remember going into a health food store with a friend and thinking, "Well, shoot… they don't have a thing to eat in this place!" Now I think that when I walk through the aisles of a regular grocery store.

Remember: *piano, piano!* Pick the three—or if that's too tough, pick just one of these items—you can eliminate today. When you're ready, come back to the list and pick another. You'll be surprised what can happen to your kitchen, your body, and your mind when you do that over the course of a lifetime.

Most disease is traceable ultimately to incorrect diet. The cure for such wrong eating is not in better drugs, nor necessarily in better restaurants, but in reclaiming our oldest right and duty, to cook for ourselves, and those we love.

— Amadea Morningstar

Cook with Abandon!

(or... Never Cook for One Meal or for One Person—Even if You're Single)

Let's start with some more encouragement.

When I was ten years old, my mother's boyfriend Tony taught me "You are what you eat." The lesson didn't take at the time—being macaroni and cheese sounded fine to me—but at least I was exposed to the concept. During college, like most students in the financial struggle, I lived on junk food. After college, working furiously to pay down my debts, I still found little time for food, so I continued with the drive-thru window and microwave model of existence.

I moved to Laguna Beach in my early twenties. There I soon befriended a neighbor who was an immigrant from Jamaica and worked as a gardener. New to the U.S. and our ways, she was still reeling from many discoveries: one being that Americans "bag da Earth and sell it for money!"—referring to potting soil. Another being the way we all stayed alive eating what we did.

Watching me microwave and choke down yet another meal, she finally said, "I'm gone cook for you and save your life!" And so she did. After work, I would go to her place and find beautiful Caribbean meals, fresh flowers from her garden on the table, and a book resting on my placemat that I "had to read." The first of those books on health and "proppa ways of eating" was John Robbins's *Diet for a New America*.

After reading that, "You are what you eat" sank in and stuck—and since then, I haven't stopped learning about and loving healthy eating.

Whether you're riveted on the edge of your seat to get started with some new ideas, or if you're still happy being Hamburger Helper—no worries. If you're not moved today, maybe it will happen tomorrow—or maybe as with me—it will take a few decades. Just keep reading and see what happens.

If you want to calculate how much time it takes to really cook food for a family, you'll need to remember how to do your math problems from grade school.

For example:

Breakfast usually requires 30 minutes, lunch 30 minutes, and dinner an hour, on average. On occasion, less time is required and frequently, more.

Based on those figures, that's:

$$2 \text{ (hours a day)}$$
$$\underline{x \quad 365 \text{ (days a year)}}$$
$$= \quad 730 \text{ (hours per year)}$$

What does 730 hours mean? In normal 8-hour-a-day job terms, that's 91 days of nothing but cooking. 91 days! And that is only cooking time. That doesn't include actually eating, nor the shopping and cleaning.

Is it any wonder Americans, raising families in utter isolation from any village and with mothers working, have turned to factory foods? Who wants to spend 91 days cooking even if we're not working outside the home?

Good news: As I've promised, there are ways to start reclaiming your kitchen and your family's health. Easily.

Let's start cooking with ABANDON, meaning a lot of food at once.

So you can visualize this idea in action, I'll offer illustrations with several foods and meals and show you how to very efficiently eat three nutritious, homemade meals a day.

Let's get started!

Breakfast

For breakfast, I prepare organic, pasture-raised eggs sautéed with mushrooms, spinach, green onions, and tomatoes. Sometimes a chard and kale frittata. Sometimes a carrot and curry omelet. (Neighbors are jealous when they walk by our door and smell the aroma of our breakfast floating over the street!)

Sometimes it's porridge of organic steel cut oats and quinoa (soaked overnight to speed cook time and for nutritional benefits). I add spices, fruits, and nuts like sliced dates and raisins, chopped pecans, ghee (or butter), cardamom, and cinnamon. I top it off with soymilk or raw, organic boiled milk. When there's time, I complement the porridge with eggs sautéed in turmeric and spinach.

That is truly a breakfast of champions: a complex carb full of minerals, fiber, and flavor that, according to Traditional Chinese Medicine (TCM), gives the body energy and simultaneously calms the mind. A clean protein, an iron-packed vegetable, and spices that warm the digestive system and improve circulation.

Whoa! Just typing that makes me hungry even though I just ate.

If I'm really in a hurry, it might be just a boiled egg and a scoop of leftover sweet potato.

Though they may seem complex and never feel the radiation of a microwave, almost all my meals are quick and easy to prepare.

Lunch

Lunch is almost always leftovers from dinner the night before. It might be a 5-bean chili or 10-veggie stew; chicken curry with celery, potatoes, and okra; or a fiery bowl of chili with bell peppers, celery, and carrots. On the lighter side, an avocado stuffed with chicken or tuna salad, with lightly steamed Brussels sprouts and cauliflower on the side.

Dinner

Dinner can be a whole chicken roasted with rosemary, garlic, potatoes, onions, parsnips, and carrots, with steamed greens on the side. Or seaweed in shrimp broth and green bean and tofu curry with sautéed bok choy on the side. Perhaps cumin black bean and cilantro burritos with tomato, brown rice, tomatillo salsa, and guacamole.

It may seem a daunting task to prepare such meals every day, but over time, I've found ways to not only figure out how to do it, but how to do so without living in my kitchen.

You won't prepare the same meals I do, but the approach I use to cooking can be applied to any style or cuisine. Let's look at meal preparation by ingredient group:

Vegetables

Review the meals listed above again and notice how many vegetables are included!

If I cooked each one of those meals with no prior preparation, from scratch, every time, my kitchen time would far exceed our 730 hours per year. But it doesn't.

Breakfast takes 10 minutes because I've already prepped all the ingredients before I need them.

Because it was prepared the night before, lunch is a homemade, organic meal that takes 10 minutes to heat and serve. Clean-up adds five minutes.

I cook twice the amount of food I'll need for dinner—if not three times, in which case I freeze one portion for use when I have even less time to cook. Though dinner is often the most time-consuming meal prep of the day, it still takes much less time if I've already prepped the primary ingredients in large batches before I need to use them.

Often the vegetable prep is the most time-consuming in any meal. If I had to prepare veggies from beginning to end at every meal, I'd probably stop eating veggies! It's not the manual labor, but the time and tedium of doing it three times a day.

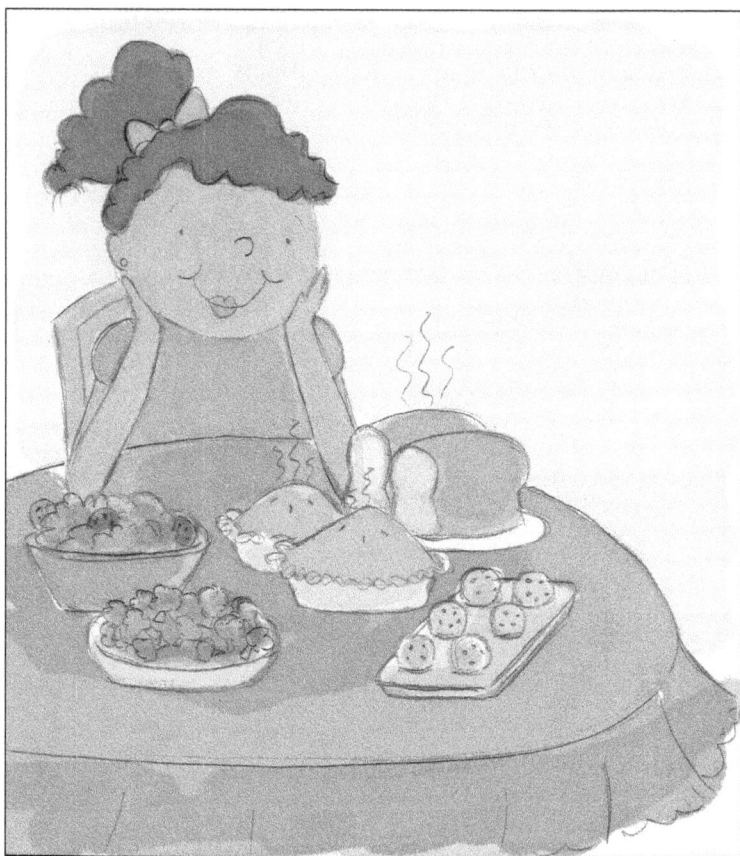

No matter what you prepare, prepare two or more at the same time.

If you are going to wash, chop, and steam broccoli, celery, and chard for dinner, wash and chop *all you have* of each. That will be a big pile of greens, but you won't use it all at one time.

Place the amount your family will eat in the steamer and the remaining veggies in containers in the fridge.

No matter what you prepare, prepare two or more at the same time.

Then, for the next two or three meals, rather than all the time of sorting, washing, and chopping, you'll just toss what's ready in a skillet and sauté with your eggs, or throw it in a steamer. Veggies in 3-10 minutes (depending on which vegetables, how large you chop them, and how soft you prefer them). *Voilà!*

If you use herbs to complement your meals (fresh rosemary, thyme, tarragon, etc.), the same approach applies. Wash and chop *all the herbs* you have at one time and store them in the fridge until you're ready to use them. The exception here is basil, which doesn't keep well once it's cut.

Eggs

Eggs are a great "cook ahead" food—and by far the easiest. Place a dozen eggs in a pan of water, bring to a boil, turn the water off, and let them sit in the hot water for 12-15 minutes. I store them in my fridge for up to four days, though some people will store them longer.

Then when you need to eat in 5 minutes, pull one out of the fridge, peel it, eat as-is, or make egg salad. If you need to eat on the run, peel it and get out the door with your perfect protein.

They are great tossed in children's lunch boxes, too. An egg, brown rice with chopped broccoli, and a piece of fruit—cheap, easy, and incredibly nutritious. It may be tough to convince your kids—at first—that they are blessed to have such a lunch, but we'll address that later. Trust me: in the last 15 years I've taught eight children ages 4-12 not only to eat what they're provided without complaint, but also to say "thank you" and to wash the dishes.

Mama don't take no mess!

Grains, Beans, and Legumes

Whole grains, beans, and legumes are great sources of nutrition and require very little prep time. It's the cook time that's the problem—unless we prepare properly.

Beans must be rinsed and soaked in a bowl of water overnight, then cooked 1-2 hours depending on which variety.

Brown and black rice (my favorites) take 5 minutes to prepare, but 50 minutes to cook. Of course most families don't have an hour to wait for rice to cook when they get home from work at 6:30 and put kids to bed at 8:00. Neither do I!

However, when I do have a full hour or two for uninterrupted kitchen time, I start the beans and the rice first—four meals' worth each!

Back to our math problems: why cook 8 cups of rice (four meals for two people) for four separate hours when you can cook four meals' worth in just one hour? Cook all 8 cups at once and store it in 2-cup containers in the fridge.

Note: Leftover rice is very easy to heat, and the texture and flavor are just as good as freshly cooked. Simply put the rice in a skillet with a small amount of oil and water in the bottom of the pan and steam it covered for a few minutes. Ditto for beans.

And if I'm going to spend an hour in the kitchen preparing rice (brown, black, basmati, jasmine, etc.), beans (black, navy, fava, etc.), and legumes (lentils, split peas, etc.) for our dinners, I can just as easily start a pot with four meals' worth of breakfast grains (oats, amaranth, quinoa, teff, etc.) *at the same time.*

The grains I eat for breakfast require 30-40 minutes cook time, so they're the perfect thing to start once the beans and rice are going.

Then, while the beans, rice, and breakfast grains cook, I wash and chop veggies and herbs.

Get the picture? It seems like a lot of multi-tasking and perhaps overwhelming, but it's really simple.

Let's break it down:

1. Add beans (that were soaked overnight) to boiling water, reduce to simmer and cook 90 minutes.

2. Add rice to boiling water (or broth), reduce to simmer, cover, and cook 50 minutes.

3. Add oats to boiling water, reduce heat, and simmer 35 minutes.

4. Wash and chop vegetables.

At the end of two hours in the kitchen, I have four meals' worth of rice, four meals' worth of beans, four meals' worth of breakfast grains, and all my vegetables prepared.

Can you see the phenomenal timesaving that comes with simply setting aside two hours to cook? The outline above doesn't completely prepare 12 meals, but it does prepare the major ingredients for those 12 meals and means that when it comes time to eat, I can make incredible meals in 30 minutes or less.

For the final touch, I make these two hours of *fun!* I listen to great music, to my foreign language lessons, or inspirational lectures. I actually look forward to these times and often my husband will join me, help with the prep work, and clean up— which makes it even more fun. *A little time for free love!*

Remember this simple lesson every time you're in the kitchen. You'll be amazed how it makes cooking something you look forward to—and that you gladly do much more often, and with better ingredients.

To your health!

Soups and Stews to the Rescue

For those who are health conscious, want to eat delicious meals, need to take them to school or work, and don't have much time—soups and stews should be your mainstay!

> In general, a soup is lighter and more liquid, and a stew is thicker and heartier.

If you follow the idea of cooking with abandon, you're going to have lots of beans, grains, and vegetables already cooked and waiting in your fridge. Whenever you're in a hurry, or whenever those pre-cooked items are on their last day and need to be used or tossed—don't throw them out—throw them in a soup!

Take a soup pot, coat the bottom with olive oil, sauté onions and your choice of spices, throw in any mix of vegetables, grains, and beans that pleases you; cover with water; and in 10 minutes you have a complete meal. If you have leftover meats, toss them in too. Chopped herbs from previous meals go in the pot in the last few minutes so their flavor is preserved (cooking herbs too long diminishes the flavor).

Essentially, open the fridge and everything goes in the pot! What could be easier?

If you have the time and desire, you can complement your meal with a fresh salad and bread, but soup alone offers complete nutrition.

Of course, there are thousands of soup recipes, which keeps things fresh and fun for the cook—and for the palate of all those eating—so try new ones all the time.

After you eat your delicious soup or stew for dinner, warm the leftovers in the morning, pour in a thermos, and send your loved ones to work and school with a complete hot, delicious lunch. Your prep time: 5 minutes!

And people say they don't have time to make their kids' lunch! Well, if you ever said that, you won't need to anymore.

Eat High ROI Staple Foods—
Yams, Potatoes, and Sea Vegetables!

Yams

You may not think so yet, but this is an exciting subject!

Sweet potatoes (or yams) have one of the highest ROIs (return on investment, or if you prefer, nutritional bang for the buck) of any food: one of the very easiest foods to prepare, delicious for even finicky eaters, and super nutritious. Oh, if only Wall Street could give us the ROI of sweet potatoes!

From a Western nutrition perspective, they are a high quality, complex carbohydrate and full of vitamins and antioxidants. From a TCM perspective, sweet potatoes benefit digestion and the kidneys (associated with strength and longevity).

As my friend (the Jamaican gardener) said when I called asking if I could still eat a sweet potato I'd cooked and left on the counter overnight: *Sweet potatoes have a life of their own!*

To prepare them: rinse, place them in a baking dish, prick with a fork a few times, and put in the oven on 375º until soft (30-60 minutes based on size). They're ready when a fork slides in easily.

To serve: cut open, put on a plate, and scoop out with a spoon—from fridge to table in 5 minutes of work.

OK, but who has 30-60 minutes to wait?

Referring back to "Cook with Abandon," to save time and have this power-packed food ready to eat whenever you're hungry, cook three or four of them and store them in the fridge in their skins or scoop out and store ready to eat.

Potatoes

Russet, Yukon Gold, red, purple, and other varieties of potatoes bring their own nutrition and tastes to the party. They can be prepared in many ways, but either baking or boiling is the fastest and easiest.

To bake: wash, cut out any green or rotting spots (ideally there won't be any—and if there are several, that potato should be tossed), place in a baking dish, and bake at 350 degrees until tender. (Again, time varies with the size of the potatoes.)

To boil: wash, chop, cover in water, and boil until soft, about 10 minutes.

Easy!

You can eat the inside mashed with herbs and butter at one meal, and then stuff the skins with a range of ingredients for the next meal. I prefer to eat the inside and skin together—the fiber helps control any glucose spike that can occur when eating carbs, and the skins are mineral-rich.

Whichever way you enjoy eating them, as with sweet potatoes: never cook one at a time—cook four or five!

A great idea for a lunch thermos: Chop potatoes with skins on, boil until soft, then mash with ghee (clarified butter) or butter. Throw in finely chopped and steamed veggies and herbs that you already have in the fridge. Add just a cup of parsley and broccoli to make them delicious and extra nutritious, stir, and in the thermos they go. A perfect lunch. If you eat meat, chop leftovers fine and toss them in the mix.

These are just a few ideas to get you going with the concept of easy, fast, nutritious, and fun food preparation. There are no real "rules" in cooking, and over time you'll find infinite ideas and combinations to build on these simple recipes.

Sea Vegetables

Why are sea vegetables in a category separate from land vegetables?

The first reason is that so many people are still unfamiliar with them (other than perhaps in sushi bars), and of those who have seen or eaten them in restaurants, far fewer prepare them at home.

The other reasons are that they offer incredibly dense nutrition—containing 10-20 times the minerals of land vegetables,[11] they're fast and easy to prepare, and unlike their cousins on land, they can keep for a *long time* in the cupboard.

> My first exposure to sea veggies was not at the kitchen table, but scuba diving in the Pacific Ocean. I was riding a current about 40 feet deep and headed straight into a kelp forest. It was like a dream. Rays of light were streaming down from the surface and shining on the kelp; the current carried me through the forest like a leaf on the wind. Sometimes a positive association can increase our appreciation for a food!

11. Paul Pitchford, *Healing with Whole Foods: Asian Traditions and Modern Nutrition*, 3rd Edition (Berkeley, California: North Atlantic Books, 2002), p. 580.

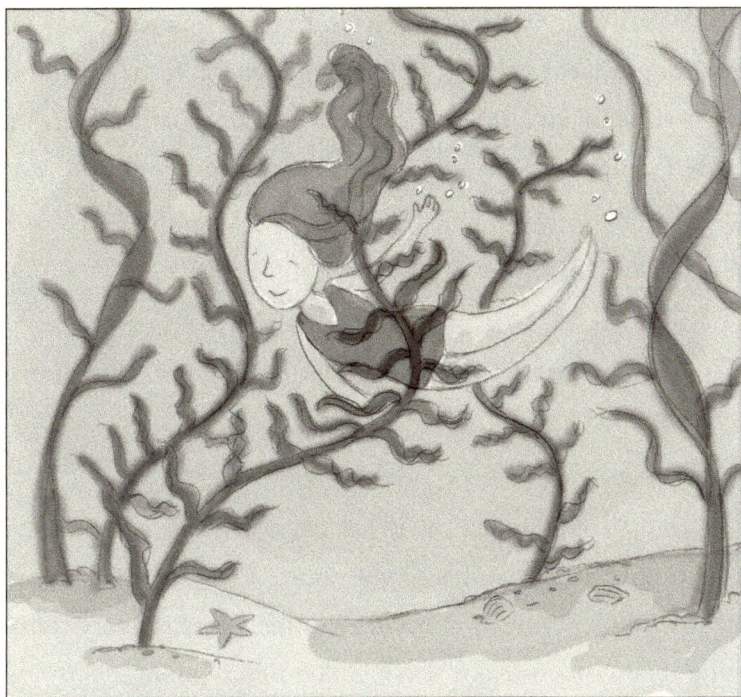

Swimming through a kelp forest is a quick way to fall in love with seaweed.

Back on dry ground, vegetables—especially organic—can get seriously expensive, which makes it particularly discouraging to open a fridge and see half of them wilting before you've had time to prepare them. (But now you know what to do with them. Quick! Make a soup before they go bad.)

More happy news! That won't happen with sea veggies— also called seaweed.

Day or night, today or two weeks from now, that seaweed you bought last week will be there ready to give an enormous boost to your vitamin and mineral intake. Further, they are known to have special properties, like the ability to bind with and eliminate heavy metals and radioactive material in the body.[12] No small benefit in our modern world.

If those reasons aren't compelling enough to eat seaweed, here are some more!

Though it is rarely discussed from this angle, seaweed is very important for women to consume. Why women? We have slightly different nutrition needs than men, one primary reason being that we menstruate. Losing blood every month is natural, but we must eat in a way that restores what was lost. Our modern diet of processed foods does not do that sufficiently, and many people end up with "blood deficiency."

Western medicine finds this situation difficult to diagnose, and even when blood tests show adequate nutrients, according to TCM, a person may still have blood deficiency—which leads to many problems including:

---

12. Pitchford, p. 581.

- Anxiety

- Irregular, light, or short periods

- Fatigue, especially before or after the period

- Numbness or tingling in the extremities

Insufficient blood means that the blood can't circulate well, which leads to "blood stagnation," which in turn creates a whole new set of problems we don't want! (Just think of a stagnant creek and you get the picture.)

There are many foods that "build blood," and seaweed is one such group.

I can already hear the questions—I asked the same ones when I first encountered seaweed.

Where do you buy it, which varieties do you eat, and how do you prepare them?

There are many types of seaweed, each with unique properties. The good news is: You can't go wrong with any one you choose. Some of the most common:

- Nori: Flat dark green sheets

- Kombu: Also called kelp—the stuff you see floating in beds on the ocean surface

- Dulse: A deep red color

- Sea Palm: It looks like it sounds—like tiny palm fronds

- Wakame and Arame: Usually sold as dark green strips

Since they are sold dried, to prepare any of them (other than nori) first soak in a bowl of water to reconstitute. Toss that water out, and you have your sea veggie. You can chop it fine and eat "as-is," toss it in soup, or mix in salads with land veggies.

To get you going, I'll tell you my two favorite, easy ways to eat seaweed:

Eggs Wrapped in Nori

Prep time: 5 minutes

Cost: 15-30¢ (depending on the type of egg purchased)

Ingredients:

Eggs

Nori

Butter or oil

Toasted sesame oil (optional)

Scramble or fry an egg in butter or oil, wrap in a dry sheet of nori, drizzle with toasted sesame oil (optional), and chow down! This is so delicious, so easy to make, and so nutritious, I eat it several times a week for breakfast—and say a prayer of gratitude that I get to!

Mixed Seaweed Soup

Prep time: 10 minutes

Cost: varies with veggies, but less than $1 per serving

Ingredients:

Broth (recipe on page 91) or water

Choice of seaweed, veggies, and herbs

Take any broth or plain water, toss in any mix of rehydrated seaweed, any mix of veggies (sprouts, greens, carrots, etc.), any mix of herbs (cilantro and parsley are excellent), and simmer for a few minutes. A veritable primordial soup awaits to give you new life.

If you like, stir in a tablespoon of miso (fermented soybean paste—an ancient food) after you remove the soup from the heat. It adds great flavor and more nutrition.

Because there is so much nutritional deficiency in the standard American diet, seaweed's value can't be underestimated. We will greatly benefit from adding it to the menu at least a few times a week, if not every day.

It can be found at any health food store, including the big chain health food stores. Because of issues affecting the oceans, I look for seaweed harvested from the U.S. Pacific Coast or Iceland. BUT, I would eat seaweed from whatever source I could find if choices were limited.

If I haven't convinced you on seaweed yet, here's my last try—and for any stragglers to the party, this should do the trick! Seaweed has been revered in Asian culture for centuries for its ability to enhance beauty, especially affecting skin, hair, and nails.

If Any... Less Meat, More Bones

Much attention has been given by the media in the last few decades to the sordid condition of meat production in the U.S. and around the world.

For those interested, the person who has covered the subject with great depth, knowledge, love—and first-hand experience—is an author already mentioned: John Robbins, author of *Diet for A New America*, *The New Good Life*, *No Happy Cows*, and others.

Robbins' legacy was to inherit the Baskin Robbins billion-dollar biz, but, unwilling to pursue a career and fortune in something he knew to be so harmful to the health of people, animals, and the entire earth, he dedicated his life and work to educating people about the cruelty and harm in factory farming.

I read *Diet for a New America* in 1994, and never looked back. It changed the way I ate then, now, and for the rest of my life. Initially I stopped eating all meat. And though I believe now—for my body and lifestyle—a little meat is beneficial, if I didn't have access to the meat that I do, I would never eat any.

This subject is discussed with the same passion as religion, and my thought (as with religion and spirituality), is that individuals must study, pray, and weigh the consequences of their decisions and actions themselves—not under pressure or force from others.

When I moved to Northern California, I found easier access to what I believed were some of the best farms in the U.S. and a way to eat meat with which I felt happy and healthy. I drove to farms, met ranchers, helped tend to their animals during my visits, saw the ranchers' hearts heavy at slaughter times, and saw the *respect* with which the animals were treated while alive.

The small number of special animals on these few, special farms roam on huge open hills covered in fluffy green grass and spend their days—all their days—wandering in the sun and grazing. The great, vast majority of cows are (in my view) tortured and miserable (including those advertised as "happy"). Even if only for reasons of self-preservation, I wouldn't eat most meat or meat "products."

Another thing I've changed is *the way* I eat meat. When I do eat an animal, I eat one—three times!

Three times?

When I was a kid, meaning in the 70s, I remember going to the grocery store with my mother and seeing the meat department. In it were men who looked "scary" to me, because they wore aprons covered in blood. However, they were butchers, and they butchered animals—meaning they cut animals into all the various sections of muscle, organs, and bones—and then presented them for sale. There were rows of hearts, brains, eyes, tongues, kidneys, necks, and tails—every part was available and used.

Today in the U.S., we scarcely see an organ or bone, and if we do, we wouldn't know what to do with it, other than throw it away.

Throw it away?

That's a terrible waste for more than one reason.

- First, those animals lose their lives for our gain (or our loss, depending on your position), and we're going to take a few bits and throw out the rest?

Initially, I was surprised when I shopped in a large health food grocery. It had row after row of organic, 100% grass-fed beef; row after row of organic, free-range chicken; and row after row of wild-caught fish. "Do you have any bones?" I asked. "No, we don't carry them." No fish bones, no chicken bones, no cow bones.

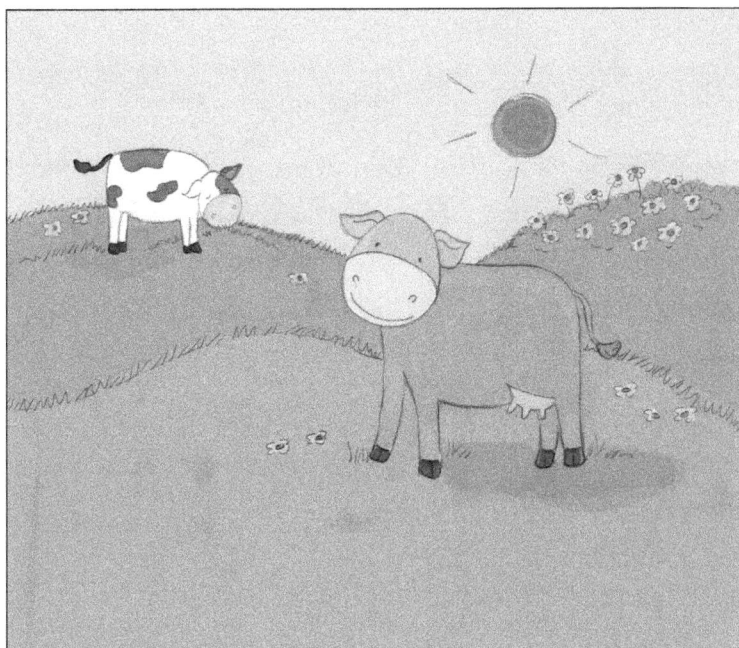

Here's an image we're sold. To find a ranch that truly treated animals well and where I could buy meat directly from that rancher, I searched for weeks and drove for hours. However, I don't believe there is a single grocery store where meat can be purchased where the animals lived "happy" or natural lives.

What are they doing with all the bones? Grinding them and putting them in dog food? Processed food for people? Or who knows what else? Not one butcher has been able to tell me exactly what's happening to all those bones and organs.

- The second reason it's a terrible shame to toss out bones and organs is that it's an enormous waste of nutrition.

Interestingly, according to many schools of medicine and nutrition, those major parts we're tossing out—the bones and organs—offer unique and important nutrients not offered by the muscles. Those parts are included in the daily cuisine of people around the world—and used to be in the U.S. But they aren't, or at least not often, in our grocery stores anymore. Further, the people working behind the counters aren't really butchers anymore, either. They receive ready-cut pieces by the millions from factories.

So back to the idea that I eat one animal three times. When I eat chicken, I pay a huge price for it relative to the average chicken in the grocery store, but I'm paying *less per serving* than most people.

I've seen where the chickens live: in sprawling, grassy meadows and hen houses that smell fresh and clean—because they are. I've seen what they eat: grubs, worms, and insects, supplemented with organic feed. I've seen how they look while alive: gorgeous.

When I then buy one to eat—maybe some will see it as a ridiculous or romantic notion or justification, by those who abstain—I want to pay respect to the animal by leaving nothing to waste.

The first time I prepare a chicken, I remove the organs and bake the chicken whole. The first meal is prepared with chicken meat—a whole chicken will yield 6 servings with the amount I use (adequate for my nutritional standards but not huge chunks as a main or only dish).

For the second round, I prepare the organs, sautéing the liver to serve in a salad of field greens or including the organs in a soup. For those with blood deficiency, this is highly recommended food by TCM.

The third time I prepare the chicken is by simmering all the bones—and if they are included when I buy it, the head and the feet—for 24 hours to prepare a broth to drink as-is or to use in further soup preparation. Bone broth prepared in this way is considered a healing and strength-giving food around the world. It would be considered gluttonous and crude to throw out the bones. (If we come to see it this way, we can forgive ourselves for not having seen or known anything different before.) This broth will be used in up to 10 servings of soup.

So it's time for one of those math problems.

If I pay $25 for the best chicken that I buy directly from a farm (meaning, it had the most natural experience possible given that it was to be used ultimately as food), and cook it 3 times, yielding 20 servings, how much does each serving of organic chicken cost?

$1.25 per serving.

Now, if I paid $10 per whole chicken raised in a battery cage and treated with extreme cruelty (in my view) and cooked it once, served each family member an equal share—yielding 4 servings—and then threw away the rest, how much does each serving cost?

$2.50 per serving.

People often say, *I can't afford organic foods.* I sympathize with their feelings, but the math as I work it out above says *yes they can!*

Implementing the Less Meat, More Bones concept, we get 4x the servings from one animal, we pay 50% of the price per serving, and we get much more nutrition. This all means that we would only need to raise and slaughter 25% of the number of animals we do currently.

I don't know the math formula for that, but I can assure you that if we consumed only 25% of the meat we do now, trees, air, water, our health, and the animals would all benefit—and we'd be heading in an exciting new direction!

If the concept of cooking with bones and organs is new to you, I'm going to give you two ideas here to get you started.

At first, it may seem gross or creepy to hold or even look at these parts. I can empathize. I was freaked out when I first held a chicken liver in my hand.

All I can tell you is: If you choose to eat meat, this should be no more or less creepy than looking at or eating the muscle—it's just a matter of what we're accustomed to.

Bone Broth

Prep-time: 10-15 minutes

This is where a crock-pot comes in handy.

Ingredients:

Any bones

Any vegetables

First, place the bones in a pot of boiling water on the stove. Remove them after a few minutes and throw out the water. (This is called "blanching" the bones in recipes—and it makes for a clearer broth.)

Place the bones in the crock-pot, cover with fresh water, and cook on low 12-24 hours. (Slow, long cooking helps not only the flavor, but it pulls more of those important minerals from the bones.)

After you've cooked the bones, add a few handfuls of prepped veggies from the fridge and cook on low for another two hours.

Then drain the broth, and strain through cheesecloth if you want a clear broth. (This step is optional.)

You can drink this as a light soup, or you can use it as your base for any soup, stew, or chili—or in place of water when cooking rice and/or beans.

You will be shocked at how much more delicious any soup recipe is with this type of broth. Further, it will be power-packed with more nutrition.

Chicken Liver Salad

Prep-time: 10-15 minutes

Ingredients:

Chicken livers

Green onions

Olive oil

Sesame oil (optional)

Greens / Lettuce

Wash livers in water and dice.

Dice 2-3 green onions

Sauté liver and green onions in olive oil until cooked through (a few minutes).

Toss in toasted sesame oil after cooking (optional) and mix with any lettuce and greens.

We'll conclude this section with a story about my first, special encounter with chicken bones and how far one could stretch one chicken in meal preparation.

When I was in Paris for the first time in 1990, I stayed at the long-famous and since-gone bookstore, *Shakespeare and Company*, with the owner, George Whitman—the grandson of our beloved American writer, Walt Whitman.

I'd read about the bookstore before going to France and, adoring the work of Walt Whitman, I decided to see if I could meet George.

The bookstore was packed with books. Let's elaborate on "packed": floor to ceiling against every wall, and stacked four feet high and deep on every table. The store was three stories high—and every room a pile and maze of books. The kitchen, the bathroom: floor to ceiling books.

In the corners of the rooms—framed by books, were mattresses. On these mattresses slept travelers from far and wide who needed a place to crash—for free—in one of the most expensive cities in the world. As you can imagine, it was a young and rag-tag group, but an interesting crowd—essentially the same faces you'd see in a youth hostel.

When I approached the building the first time, an elderly gentleman stood at the door and instructed me to go in and buy a book. I guessed I'd found George, and I had. I introduced myself and started to ask him a question when he cut in,

"How many nights are you staying with us in the bookstore?"

I explained that a relative of my boss had given little-broke-me an apartment to stay in for the month—a 20 million-Franc (US$4-5 million) apartment according to the nosy neighbors—that was their family Paris-for-the-weekend crash-pad, and that I was just happy to meet him and shop for books.

He cut in again, "Well, let's start with a week stay and take it from there."

When George speaks, Allie listens. But I decided to stay one night.

One night at the *Shakespeare and Company* bookstore with George Whitman and a collection of fellow broke travelers. It sounded fun! Painted in gold over the entrance was a banner: *Be kind to strangers lest they be angels in disguise.*

He explained the rules: Anyone who needed a place could stay, but for every night they stayed, they had to read one book and do one chore.

I said I understood and asked if he'd be so kind as to select my book. That is how I came to read the utterly grim *The Idiot* by Dostoyevsky.[13] A deal's a deal.

When I woke the next morning on my lumpy, dirty mattress, I asked George for my chore assignment. He said, "I have a writer coming today, and I need to make a soup for him. Take the chicken bones you'll find in the kitchen, remove the meat, and put it in the soup pot."

That sounded easy enough, but when I got to the kitchen, there was only a dry skeleton of a chicken on the counter

---

13. Why, why, why haven't we advanced from the unquestioning admiration (and required reading) of the literature of dark and dank corners of the world, written by debauched, drunken, and depressed cranks and pedophiles? And why is *Lolita* on children's summer reading lists? I'm glad I read *The Idiot*, but mainly because George told me to.

When we decide that happy literature can also merit awards, I have a nomination: Celestine Vaite, a Tahitian writer, stated in an interview that her goal was to win the Nobel Prize for literature—and I hope she does. Her trilogy, *Breadfruit, Frangipani,* and *Tiare in Bloom* is marvelous. It contains everything the old-guard requires: teenage mothers, drunkenness, brawls with machetes, oppression of the poor—but from every page stream rays of South Pacific sunshine.

I wrote to her to thank her for her work, and she wrote back, saying her next trilogy was underway. I haven't seen it yet. Celestine—I hope you're sitting at your computer right now!

that looked like it had been abandoned a week prior. I called to George, "I only see chicken bones...nothing with meat" (I guess I expected what I'd see in the U.S.—two 3-pound breasts and two 2-pound legs).

He sprang to the kitchen and lurched at the chicken. "Oh, you ri-i-ich kids! Damn it! Those bones are covered in meat! You see! You see!" he screamed, shaking the skeleton.

I guessed him to be around 80 and hadn't expected him to be so spry or passionate. I was already enamored of this old eccentric, and this was making my crush worse. I wanted to crack up laughing, but I didn't want him thinking I was an entitled little shite.

"Oh, yes, I see now!" I apologized and started to remove the minute remains of tendon and skin from the deep crevices in the bones.

"Now wipe these pans clean with this newspaper and make everything look nice."

I wondered how to wipe something clean with something dirty, but I was catching on—just move when he says to do something.

Suddenly, in a completely new tone, he said,

"I like you here. You put up with my..." and then his gaze turned to the sink.

"*WHAT IS THAT?*" he screeched. "I said to make it look nice. You don't do it like—that doesn't look nice. *Like this!*" he said scrubbing ferociously.

I decided to come out of character and call him out of his. "George, you are adorable, and I'm not buying this grouchy old man routine, either—or at least not entirely."

He answered, "You said you're from Texas? You're not a Texan. You're Dostoyevsky's Anastassya."

"I'm leaving today, George."

"Well, then you'll come back in a few days, won't you?"

"Yes," I said, planting a kiss on his cheek.

"Well, before you go, pull out a clean towel from the laundry for the writer."

Then I made another mistake.

"A big one or one of these small ones?" I asked.

His eyes bulged.

"*A SMALL ONE!* Big towels are *ridiculous* and should all be cut into six pieces! Well... maybe the writer likes big ones... leave out a big one. Ri-i-i-ich kids!"

I thanked him, blew a kiss, and turned to leave.

He called, "You said you'd be here for tea at 4:00 tomorrow. Will you be?"

"Yes, George. 4:00."

The Family that Cooks Together, Stays Together

There are many families who enjoy cooking together, but the more common picture one sees today is: Mom or dad rushes to microwave a plastic package, bake something that was frozen in a box, or serve something purchased on the way home from work at a drive-thru window. Often, kids have already microwaved something for themselves before the parents arrive home, so family members eat separately.

Well, no wonder.

If the job is left to one person, and that person has a huge list of other responsibilities for the day, what else can they do?

If the family has not come to an agreement to divide the jobs of breadwinning and bread baking, then it is ideal if everyone chips in to help cook, or family members take turns at the hearth.

Most fun is when the family gathers together and shares in the preparation. For example: Put on some great music, Mom works the stove, Dad is *sous-chef*, and the kiddos wash veggies and help clean.

My husband and I work together in the kitchen all the time, and we've come up with some pretty goofy rituals that we adore. I know the sure way to get him away from a screen and in the kitchen to work his Malaysian-cuisine magic with me is to pull out his *Star Wars* apron. I mean, I like *Star Wars*, too, but my husband—suddenly he's a kitchen Jedi in that apron. No way I can get him off the stove. I like wearing different aprons—my baby's favorite is the one with the bunnies on it—but aprons don't have quite the same effect on me.

Further, music is a must. Again, we developed some really fun rituals. We listen to almost every genre and language of music, but in the kitchen it's usually songs we like to sing with. The collection includes anything by Fred Astaire, Billie Holiday, the Carpenters, Neil Diamond, and most of the musicals from the last 50 years. (Mama does love the hip-hop and Euro house, but that's not our family-time music.)

Try these rituals or think of your own. If you come up with really good ones, I'd love to hear about them. See if you can't find a way to get your groove back at the hearth and if you don't look forward to—and love—time in the kitchen!

AT HOME

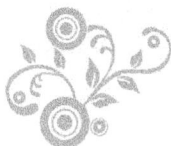

Simple, free, and beautiful ideas that anyone can implement—right now—in their home to create:

- *Better health*

- *More happiness*

- *And tons of love*

We spend hours in the kitchen (even if we prepare processed foods), yet we spend many more hours in the rest of our house.

How do we spend that time? How do we treat our dwelling, our family members, and ourselves in those precious hours—waking and sleeping—in our homes?

With the pace of our lives in this society and era, many of us spend that time in a frenzied race to get meals down, kids' homework done, homes cleaned, clothes and dishes washed, and find enough time to crash in bed. Even for those of us whose pace is less hectic—would the words *sacred, healing, peaceful,* and *loving* come to mind when you think of your time at home?

For people who express their faith within a building—for those who go to church, synagogue, temple, or martial arts schools and yoga studios to express and share their faith or life pursuits with others—consider the way you approach your time there, the feeling you have when you walk in the door, and (hopefully) the feeling you have when you see the leaders in your organization and fellow members.

The words *sacred, healing, peaceful,* and *loving* probably do come to mind when contemplating our "holy" times.

What if we felt that way—even if only for a few moments a day—in our homes?

What if we gave the same attention and value to sacred moments—to just ourselves and our family members—sitting in our living room?

What if bedtime became a holy sacrament?

Some might laugh, but just imagine…

- How you'd feel driving home from school, work, or errands if you knew that you would be greeted by loving faces, people having fun and working together toward common, worthy goals.

- If every day after work you entered a place where you felt *peaceful* and *safe* (those feelings that give meaning to life and make all the challenges worthwhile).

- If you spent the first minutes upon waking and the last few minutes before you entered that mysterious other-world called "sleep"—in which we all live part-time and rarely discuss—with loving, calming rituals.

Whether or not you already feel peaceful and sacred with your family members in your home, here are a few ideas that will assure more fun, peace, and joyful moments with them in the most sacred building in which you spend time—your home.

As with the ideas in "Free Love at the Hearth," it doesn't matter if you don't like or don't incorporate all of these ideas in your daily life. Even in you chose just one of my ideas, or if one of my ideas inspires your own new idea to implement, your life will be richer and more peaceful—and isn't that what we all want!

Wake Up Smiling

Vacations are too few, too far-between, too expensive, and too short. When I lived abroad, Europeans would ask me why Americans were so ignorant of the world around them.[14] I would answer with what I believe is one of the reasons (shortcomings in the education system not to be addressed here) and likely the only legitimate reason:

They do not have enough vacation time or money to ever leave their country.

In the U.S., most of us have two weeks of vacation each year. Ten days out of 365! That alone should be a clear explanation, but let's elaborate.

---

14. Americans are brilliant in many ways, but geography and world events are certainly not a strong point. For one tiny and horrible example: upon my return from a trip to Europe, an acquaintance of mine—college grad and intelligent—asked me how long it took me to drive from London to Germany. a.) She thought London was a country, and b.) she didn't know about the tunnel under the channel—she thought England was physically a part of continental Europe.

Take the average mom, dad, and two-kid family. If they're earning $45,000 per year, how much disposable income will they have to spend on vacation? Further, since the U.S. is geographically isolated from other countries (and even Canada and Mexico require long and expensive planes trip for most of us), how much of their ten free days will they want to spend traveling? Finally, if they only have two weeks to rest and recharge, how refreshing is it to:

- Spend $2,000–$3,000 on tickets to travel internationally (Summer rates, when kids are out of school, can be double that or more for four tickets).

- Spend $2,000–$3,000 on accommodations and meals.

- Spend one full day traveling, two-days jet-lagged, and a second full day travelling to return home, and then another two days jet-lagged?

To spend up to 10% or more of our gross income to spend two days on a plane, four days exhausted, and a few days frantically running around trying to get our "money's worth" and actually see the place we worked so hard to see… that's not a vacation! It's stressful and it's a drag! No wonder Americans succumb to Disney theme parks as their only travel destination. (I enjoy Disneyland once every decade or two, but you see the point.)

Well, there's probably not a lot most of us can do to change that situation—at least immediately—but we can bring a little "vacation" to our everyday lives.

How do we greet people when they return from vacation, especially if they've gone to a new and mysterious place all alone? Hopefully with hugs, kisses, flowers, and a lively discussion about their adventure during a welcome-home meal.

How do we greet one another in our home when we wake from sleep—the most mysterious journey we ever take?

All too often it's with a grunt, a push to get to the bathroom first, a rush to eat something made of cardboard from the microwave (if even that), then flying out the door and racing to school or work.

Ay, yay! That's a nightmare.

No wonder people queue up for double jolts of adrenal-draining caffeine—they need something to get them going and feeling "good."

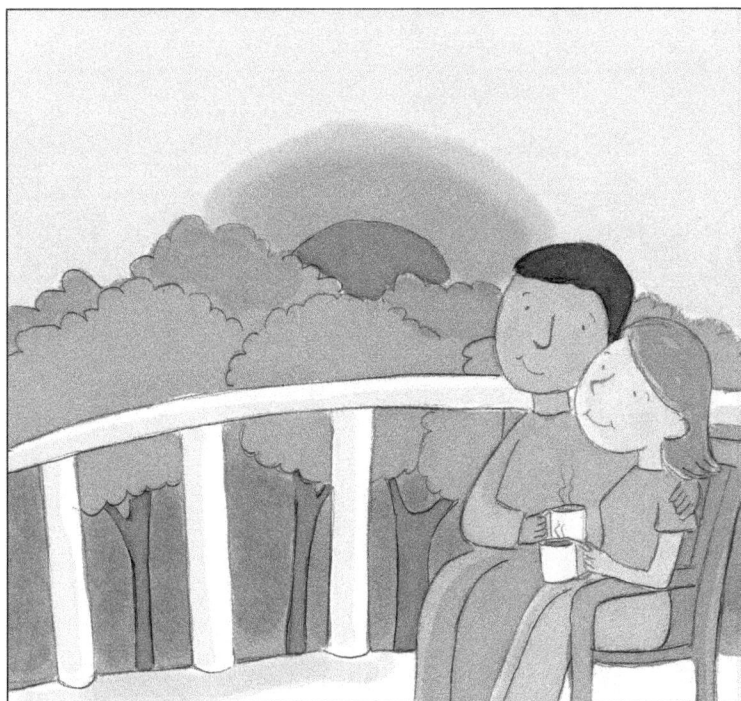

We can look forward to the alarm ringing when we create early morning rituals.

We can do better than that! And if we do, we can change the course of our days and our lives.

What if instead we set the alarm for 30 minutes earlier? That might mean we go to bed 30 minutes earlier (which many of us could do with just a little discipline), or it might mean getting 30 minutes less sleep per night. (In most instances, the small sacrifice will be well worth the perceived loss.)

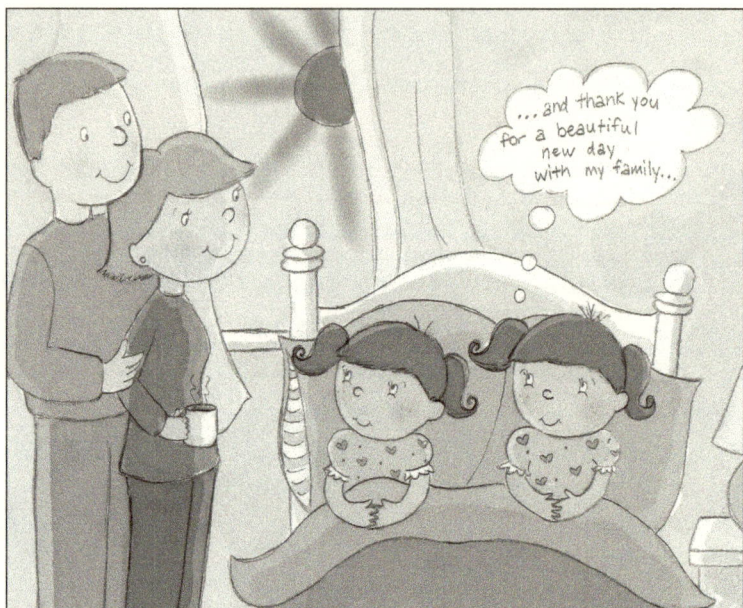

The way we start our morning can dictate the mood and direction of the day.

With that new 30-minute window, we could:

- Snuggle a few minutes in bed with our lover (remember when we called our spouse our lover?) and/or our children.

- Talk about our wild, fascinating, fun, or scary dreams.

- Say a prayer of gratitude, silently or out loud together for the blessings of the day and our lives.

- Get out of bed for 5-10 minutes of stretching together.

- Put on our robes, make our favorite tea or beverage, and sit on our front porch, balcony, terrace, in the back yard, or... if it's the only place available, on a little folding chair on the sidewalk!

Dawn (dusk and midnight, too) is a magical time, and a few minutes of calm with a warm beverage watching a sunrise... it sets a delightful pace for the day.

I saw people by the hundreds do this in the little alleys of China in the evening before bed. There on the sidewalk of the busiest streets you'd see people pull out folding chairs, tables, even hammocks (!) and either socialize, chill-out with a beverage, or just sit and watch the evening unfold. By about 10:00 p.m., they'd all be gone, and the sidewalks would quiet down. It's a lovely way to begin or end the day.

Try this every day for a week. You'll be hooked by the magic of the morning!

- Make a delicious and nutritious meal in a few minutes and share it together. (See Part 1 for breakfast ideas.)

Hear me now... believe me later. If you did all of those things in the morning, you'd feel refreshed, powerful, happy, peaceful, and ready to take on the day. Your family bonds would deepen, you would look forward to waking up (rather than dreading the alarm), and your health would benefit in a dozen ways.

Every morning can feel like waking up on vacation, so let's reclaim this precious time with our families!

(And if we'd like to beef up our knowledge of geography, we can pull out a world atlas over breakfast!)

Let's Groom Each Other

Whoa! Did she say, "*Groom* each other?"

I sure did.

A daily activity in the animal kingdom—and something we pay strangers to do for us all the time. We pay for haircuts, blow-drys, hair dos, massages, manicures, and pedicures. We even have strangers wax our bodies, including our… *genital area!*

If we're paying strangers to do these things, and we all think they feel very good (waxing, excluded), why don't we do that for our family members? It's fun, free, nurturing, and if we want it to be… it can be very sexy.

I knew a housewife, without children at the time, who was a night owl but also loved to sleep in. And I mean, *this lady could sleep!* She wouldn't get out of bed until noon many days. However, every single morning, she would get up early with her husband to blow dry his hair before he left for work, then go back to bed.

The story sounds a little funny, but what man wouldn't feel like a king having his wife wake early every morning to massage his head and neck while drying and coiffing his hair?

That may not be for everyone, but at least some form of physical care and contact would be on everyone's wish list, and not just the adults.

When I was very young, maybe seven or eight years old, one of my mother's friends—when visiting during the evenings—would come to my room and talk, or we'd go somewhere and "hang out."

One night she gave me a talk about taking vitamin C and eating oranges.

One night she showed me sketches she'd done that week.

One night we sat in her car and watched a lighting storm together from the safe haven of the garage.

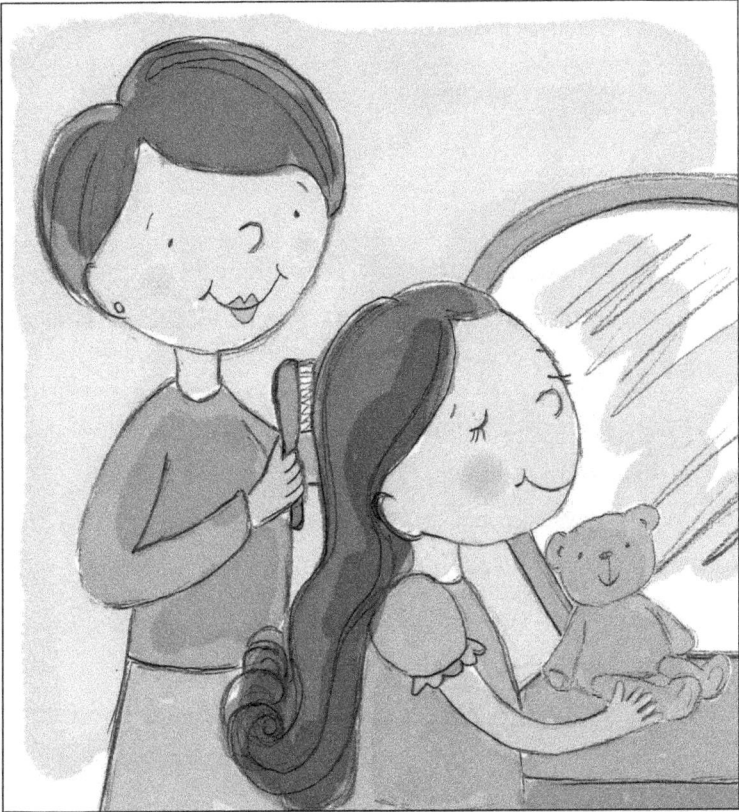

Rituals such as brushing each other's hair before bed offer time for warm, loving conversation and fun.

Every time she visited, she'd explain to me that it was healthy to brush the scalp and hair to the end, 100 strokes before bedtime each night. She would brush her long, straight hair to demonstrate and then brush mine.

(This was in the 70s. She was an artist and a "hippie." I thought she was beautiful and that everything she did was groovy.)

It felt wonderful, and not just physically. I felt special, loved, and to this day I feel that charm when recalling those brief moments with her.

I believe this was common at some time in history—before we all rushed to our separate screens before bedtime, when parents (usually mothers, but some fathers, too), brushed their children's hair and helped them groom.

Surely there are many people who do groom each other, but what if we made the effort to put a little more attention, a little more love, and a little more *intention* into caring for one another in these simple ways?

At the time, they may seem like just another part of the daily routine, but over the course of the years and a lifetime, these rituals will prove to be some of the most intimate and meaningful moments you have shared.

Call a Robe Day

One day when my husband and I were first married, we looked down at about 3:00 in the afternoon and recognized that we were both sitting in our lawn chairs, tea in hand, in bathrobes that we'd put on when we first woke up at 8:00.

We'd been so terribly busy doing nothing but relaxing that we'd forgotten to get dressed! That was a first, but not a last.

From that day forward, we decided that at certain intervals, or whenever either of us called one, we would take a robe day. Granted, this has become more challenging with an infant—and sometimes it's just a "robe hour," but however long we have, we stay in our robes, we recline and lounge, we take long baths, lie in the sun, or just sit wherever we find ourselves.

This can be better than a day at the spa, you don't need an appointment, and it's free!

All for One and One for All

In general, this is the section that will make the mamas cheer—though the papas and the children will likely boo at first, but not for long.

Household upkeep and chores should be a family commitment—not one person's commitment (or even worse, no one's commitment).

A friend of mine who works as a nanny came to my house one day with her eyes puffy and watering, coughing, and generally looking miserable. I asked what was wrong.

She said, "Oh, nothing's wrong. The family I work for had me dust and vacuum their son's room today—and since it hadn't been done since the last time I did it before I left for college seven months ago, it was pretty bad."

I said, "They leave their baby in a room that's never cleaned or dusted?"

She replied, "Oh, he's not a baby. He's 14 years old."

I was grossed out. I asked, "If he's 14, why isn't he dusting his room himself?"

She said, "The mother wants him to, but she can't get him to do it."

Did you groan like I did when you read that?

Yuck-o!

Every family has its own style of housekeeping and discipline, and below you'll read mine. I believe it accomplishes the goal of teaching discipline, self-respect, and respect for the family, along with being fun (which certainly helps).

For me, there's no such thing as "I can't get him to do it" when we're talking about a minor. I believe it is our duty as parents to teach children responsibility, discipline, and to value their ability to contribute to the family's goals and life together.

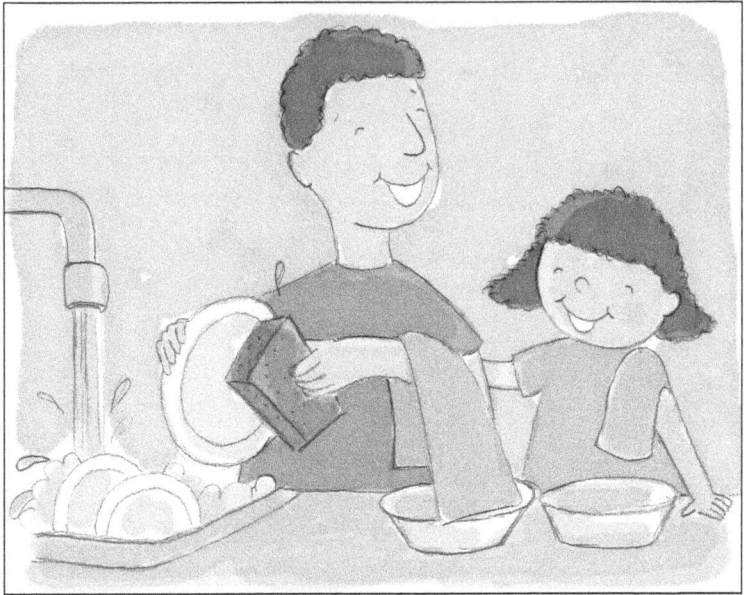

Chores are fun and easy when done together. Family members can take turns. One night Suzie helps Dad, and...

I prefer not to raise my voice, and spanking may or may not have its place and I'd rather avoid that, too. The tool I prefer to work with is the mind—and children's minds are perfectly able to comprehend, assimilate, and use the information I give them at very early ages. (Recall the children in Honduras I discussed earlier. Those children were doing—with skill—at three years the things we often fail to teach our children until they're... well... not even children any longer, if ever.)

I teach the children in my life (not only my own, but nieces, nephews, and any child who stays in my home) how to make

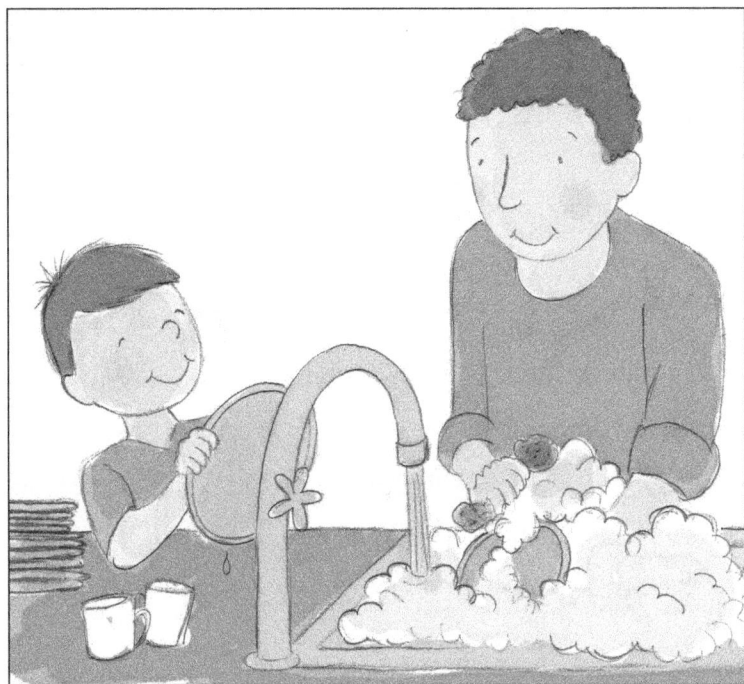

...the next night, Johnny helps Dad.

their beds, pick up their rooms, wipe down the bathroom after they use it, and clean dishes. The more time they spend with me, the more they'll know about keeping house, cooking healthy food, washing their clothes, and even grooming themselves.

We make lists, we put on good music, and then we get *busy!* Chores, when done with focus and regularly, do not require much time—and a job well done merits such rewards as going to the beach, hiking in the mountains, or playing in a park.

However, chores left undone, done poorly, or done grumbling and complaining—those earn a day sitting at home—without TV, movies, or games—until the chores are completed.

It's that simple.

I don't "make" children do anything. However, they certainly don't make me—*the adult*—do anything. Using my time and precious family time, to reward someone who's failed to make their contribution to the family dwelling—that's not in the cards.

Those new to this concept might think this leads to day after day of a dirty house, groundings, and miserable moods.

Not in the least.

Most children get the message that this is the plan (and the only plan) the first time we discuss the rules. They know that I mean what I say and that if they don't do their chores I absolutely won't do what they desire later, even if I really want to go to the beach, park, or hiking that day myself.

One Thanksgiving I had the entire family to my house for dinner. My two nephews, 14 and 10, were living with me at the time. The 14-year-old knew the routine (he'd been visiting me regularly since he was born, so he knew the deal all along) and would happily and quickly complete his job, then move on to whatever fun the day offered. The 10-year-old, stubborn by nature, needed a little more time to understand the lesson.

I asked him to vacuum while I was cooking. He turned to me with serious sass in his face and voice and said,

"Why should I?"

I replied, "You certainly don't have to. However, I have limited free time. I work to pay for this house you live in, to buy groceries, and now to cook this beautiful food for you. If I need to vacuum, too, then that cuts into grocery shopping or cooking time. If you'd prefer I don't make food for you, I'll vacuum and you can sit around—hungry."

He vacuumed—and did a nice job at that.

Again, it takes resolve, but it's that simple.

But what if he'd protested and decided not to vacuum?

No argument. No yelling. No problem.

He would have sat in his room while we enjoyed a lovely Thanksgiving feast together. Smart kids (and almost all of them are extraordinarily clever) get the lesson the first time. The slower or more stubborn might require a few days of missed trips to the beach, to the park, watching a movie with the family, or a ride to a friend's house in order to get the message—but stand firm. They'll get it sooner than later. (This is naturally assuming we're dealing with a child who is generally healthy. The exception is if a child is neglected or disturbed. Then different methods of teaching and learning may be required.)

Once they're on board, they'll often initiate their contribution before you start cleaning, cooking, or whatever the day's household activity is, so they can get it behind them and get on with their activity of choice.

P.S. My 10-year-old nephew—only a few months after our Thanksgiving lesson—became my advocate. When a visiting eight-year-old refused to make his bed, he encouraged the visitor, "She cooks for you and takes you to do nice things. Just hurry up and do your part for Aunt Allie's house." The underdog became a top pick!

Come Down to Earth

I have a great time asking friends: When was the last time your feet touched Earth?

People are always amused by the question. If it was recently, they always smile and tell me their happy story of walking barefoot on the beach the day before, hiking barefoot a few months back, or just walking barefoot and rolling in the grass in their backyard.

If it's been a long time, their eyes widen as they try to remember—and then realize that their feet literally haven't touched Earth since that trip to the beach three years ago!

I have an amusing barefoot story, at least in hindsight. On first moving to the Bay Area a few years ago, I lived right off the Golden Gate Bridge, along a boardwalk. Between that boardwalk and my garden, I went barefoot almost every day.

One day when my husband and I were preparing for a business trip to Asia, I realized that I was late for an appointment to pick up some documents at the Chinese Consulate. I grabbed my keys and purse, jumped in the car, zoomed over the bridge, and screeched into a tiny parking space at the front door of the consulate just 15 minutes later, on time.

However, as I stepped out of my car, I had a strange feeling.

"Hmm, something's wrong."

And then I looked down and saw... bare feet!

After laughing, I realized that going back for shoes might delay the departure date for our trip, so I decided I had to get in that consulate building, barefoot or not.

I approached the policemen manning the metal detector with more than a little apprehension and said,

"On the way here, I stepped on a pop top and blew out my flip-flop! Can I please come in anyway?"

They didn't skip a beat, and with what I was sure was a counter to my comment and a game of wits, one said, "Sure. Walk on by."

I should have known. This was San Francisco! They were probably relieved I wasn't trying to get in without a bra.

The policemen weren't fazed, but I did get some funny looks from the 200 American and Chinese citizens waiting in line with me.

Even though it's not what I'd recommend, that barefoot story is a fun memory for me.

How long has it been since you had your feet in the soil, sand, or even snow? Feet were meant and made to be on Earth, but most often they've turned into delicate clubs in the synthetic shoes we force on them.

Shoes have their benefit and going barefoot has its drawbacks, but life wasn't meant to be wrapped in plastic! In some health circles, it's suggested that a life "separate" from Earth builds negative energy in the body and fragments the mind.

Some of the purported benefits of barefoot walking are:

• Receiving positive energy from the Earth and its negative ions. Negative ions, unlike what the term implies, bring the benefits of detoxifying and harmonizing the body and help regulate biorhythms.

- Calm the mind through focus and attention. Even on clean beaches, for example, we have to focus on every step to avoid stepping on shells, sea jellies, or other creatures. This kind of focus clears the mind—in fact, it's the goal of many activities like yoga, tai chi, and meditation.

- According to the precepts of Traditional Chinese Medicine, barefoot walking on grass, earth, or sand helps balance and harmonize the energy flow in the body.

Barefoot walking is just another one of the obvious things that we've all forgotten in our busy, penny-loafer-and-tennies lives.

Walk as if you are kissing the Earth with your feet.

— Thich Nhat Hahn
Peace is Every Step: The Path of Mindfulness in Everyday Life

If You Would Be So Kind, Manners Please!

Don't we all appreciate a smiling face, a kind word, a polite gesture?

We do. Yet increasingly, it's the norm to hear "dialogues" with children like this:

Adult: Nice to see you. How are you doing?

Child: Goood (an adjective, while maintaining a mouth-breathing stare at screen of choice).

Adult: Time for dinner.

Adult: Time for dinner.

Adult: Johnny, did you hear me?

Child: Yeaaah.

Adult: Are you enjoying your dinner?

Child: Uuuuh, it's OK.

Adult: What did you learn today at school?

Child: Nothing.

I grew up in Texas, and while it was already on the way out in the 70s, many people did still pride themselves on teaching children to interact with adults with polite dialogue. Even today, many people in the South teach their children to respond with "Yes, ma'am, No sir" and to address adults either with their title (Teacher Mary, Coach Tom) or with a Mr. or Ms. before either their first or last name (Mr. Andy, Ms. Smith).

I believe that teaching these small formalities and courtesies to children is a wonderful step in teaching self-respect and respect for society as a whole.

When I work with children in this capacity, I explain that we don't necessarily know if a stranger whom we're addressing is worthy of respect based on their personality or behavior, but as a reflection of *our self-respect*—and being polite people—we address anyone we encounter politely. (I don't agree with lessons of blind adherence to what a "grown up" says. Being "bigger" (an adult) never guaranteed someone knew more or was worthy of more honor than someone "smaller" (a child).

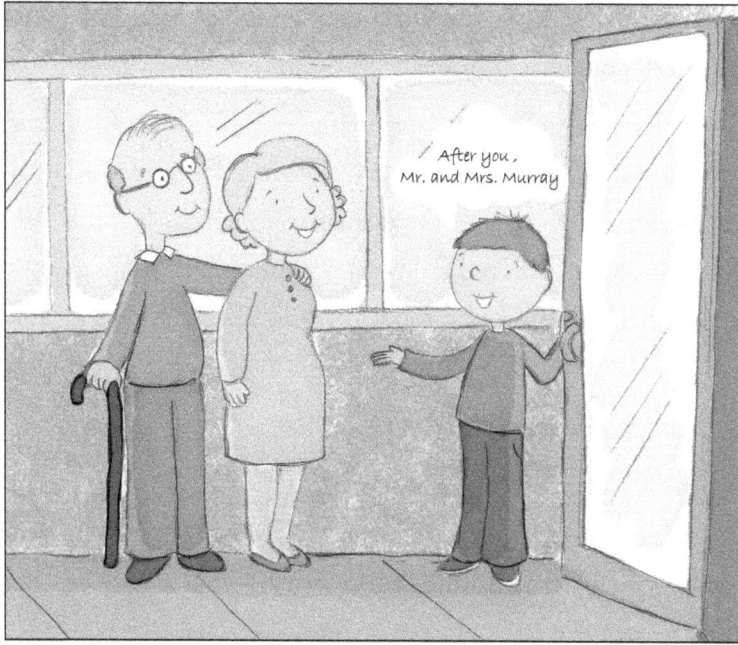

More often than not, children enjoy interacting with courtesy... once they are taught how.

I can't imagine why courtesy went out of vogue and how it became accepted and expected that children would respond to conversation with adults with sounds similar to those one hears when throwing peanuts to a caged animal—but it did.

Worse, the excuse is, "They're only kids."

I don't treat them as "only" kids—meaning, as if they were lesser beings. I treat them as people who are younger, smaller, and incredibly capable, intelligent, and innately kind[15]—even if they need guidance in how to express it.

This idea of interacting with a sunny and courteous disposition doesn't apply just to children. Don't we also love when we're shopping and the cashier is polite and helpful? Who wouldn't rather be served food in a restaurant by a smiling, polite person than someone who rudely throws our plates on the table?

This is so obvious, and yet…

We can't expect a courteous society if we don't start in our homes with basic courtesy and kindness—and what a joy it is when we do!

You never know how the smallest gesture of kindness and courtesy can change someone's day in a way they'll remember for a lifetime. With that in mind, whenever possible, let's lose the grumpy faces and grunts in lieu of words. Let's greet one another with smiles and courtesy.

Be kind whenever possible. It is always possible.

— The Dalai Lama

---

15. "Kind" is the German word for child!

Giving Thanks for Food

What does the average American family dinner scene look like? We touched on this earlier, but let's review.

From the statistics on fast food consumption, parents working late, and the general state of family and health, could this be accurate?

Mom and Dad rush home to find the kids sprawled in front of a screen and eating something they microwaved or poured from a box. The parents eat the same thing, quickly, and then crash. Or maybe Mom picks up the kids from after-school care, goes through the drive-thru window, and it's "every man for himself" when they get home.

I know that, sadly, it is increasingly acceptable to dine like this elsewhere too, but I have never witnessed this kind of meal scene in any other country. Yes, teenagers hanging in a fast-food joint and parents—from time to time—getting take out, but the standard family meal being a scene as described above… nowhere but America. And of course we all know—we even remember— it wasn't always like that.

What if, even if we're eating fast food, we all sit together at the table and turn off all screens, bells, alarms, and electronic notifications.

And what if we started our meal with a moment together in gratitude? Whether the gratitude is directed toward the Creator, toward the animals and plants that gave their lives for our nutrition, or toward the parents for earning and preparing it, it's a lovely practice to give thanks for our food.

We don't have to belong to a particular religion or any religion to sit together over a meal, hold hands, close our eyes for a moment—PAUSE and BREATHE—and say "Thank you."

Whether your concern is more with the body, the spirit, or the general state of your family relationships—all will benefit from this loving, happy practice.

Movie Night, *not* Movie Every Night

I love movies as much as anyone—maybe a lot more than most, since I haven't watched TV since 1981.

Yep, that's right. The last shows I saw on TV were *Gilligan's Island* and *I Love Lucy*—the shows that were on when I arrived home from grade school. Starting to work at Haagen-Dazs after school when I was 13 was the end of TV for me.

I've seen a few episodes of *Oprah*, I've seen *Dancing With the Stars*, and I heard of some of the big ones like *Friends*, something about bachelors and bachelorettes, another one about bimbo housewives, and... I can't think of any other names off the top of my head, but friends and family members have done their best along the way to keep me socially hip by showing me clips of this and that when I visit their homes.

When computers started coming out with DVD players, I decided that watching movies at home would be fun, and it is. I maintain a "no violence" policy and mainly watch foreign or

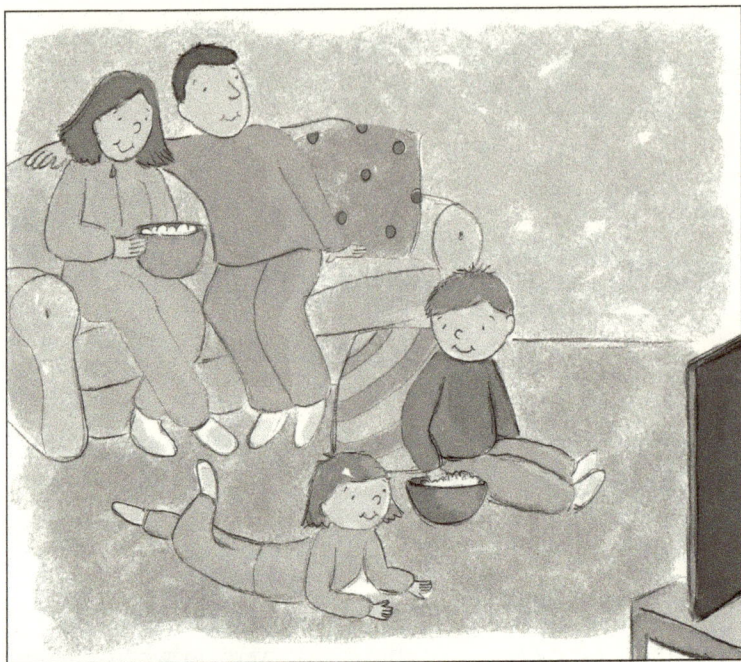

When we watch a movie once a week, rather than programming 24/7, it becomes a fun, special event.

educational films, but I'm also known to enjoy a good ridiculous comedy. Being married to a man who works on the cutting edge of technology, I've also upgraded from DVDs on the computer to a huge flat panel, 3-D Blu-Ray, streaming this and that, and some kind of tricky sound system that requires way too many outlets and wires. It's nice, but it was his idea, not mine.

No matter how much TV (or movies) we enjoy at home, we have to know that that time used is R&R time which could be used in other ways: reading with our kids, talking in the garden, taking a walk, or going for a swim together. Many of us work all day as slaves to screens. How much of our precious family time do we want to spend in front of yet another screen?

For me, the answer is: once a week—and make it a good one. Don't just flop on the sofa and click on any ol' junk, allowing advertisers to dictate that "tis the season for you to be sick."

Make it count!

Find a movie that you know is hilarious or inspiring, pile on the floor with pillows and blankets, make your favorite movie snack, hunker down with your loved ones, and relax and laugh for two hours.

Doesn't that sound fun? It sounds fun—and it is!

Bring Back the Bard

A bard was a person in medieval Gaelic and British culture who wrote or recited heroic or epic poems, often while playing a lute or harp.

Well, not many of us are practicing any aspect of that these days, and I don't think more than a few of us would want to. But if we don't do movie night every night, what will we do with that time?

One fun idea is: Let's read our favorite books aloud to each other!

Of course children love it when adults read books to them, but adults—once they've experienced it—love it, too.

Early in our relationship, my husband saw me reading *One Thousand and One Nights*, or as it's often called, *Arabian Nights*. I would read one story each night before getting ready for bed.

My hubby asked to look at it and started reading it, so we both wanted to read the one copy. We decided we would take turns reading aloud. That evolved into a tradition that we both love and to which we look forward fondly.

The story of a man named Abu Hasan who did something so "great and terrible" at his wedding that he had to leave the celebration and flee town (I'll leave it for you to discover in detail what he did, if you wish), knocked both of us out of bed. Caught so off-guard by the unexpected twist in the story, we got a case of the giggles and couldn't stop laughing and rolling around for half an hour.

In his *NY Times* article, "Some Thoughts on the Lost Art of Reading Aloud," Verlyn Klinkenborg writes, "But what I would suggest is that our idea of reading is incomplete, impoverished, unless we are also taking the time to read aloud." [16]

Once you try reading aloud with friends and family, you'll likely agree.

---

16. Verlyn Klinkenborg, "Some Thoughts on the Lost Art of Reading Aloud," *The New York Times*, May 16, 2009 (http://www.nytimes.com/2009/05/16/opinion/16sat4.html).

Git it Gone!

You know the principle of *git it gone* from our discussion in "At the Hearth." I don't reserve this mantra only for the kitchen... I use it all over the house.

A few weeks ago, a wonderful housekeeper—who just started working with us—was working in the kitchen. Suddenly, my nose and throat started burning.

From the living room I screamed, "What smells like DEATH?"

Whatever was going on, it was something unfamiliar. We don't have wretched smells in our house that burn the sense organs.

She had noticed the last time she'd been in our home that there were some areas of our stovetop that were burned, so in an act of much-appreciated initiative, she brought a chemical scouring powder to scrub it off.

I shouted, "Git it gone!"

She now knows that initiative is highly appreciated—poisonous chemicals are not.

A couple decades ago, before I'd embarked on my study of health and nutrition, I actually liked the odors of cleaning chemicals. I liked the cloud of toxins blowing in the cleaning products aisle at the grocery stores. I even told my staff in my housecleaning business—and it was true—that if we cleaned people's homes and they couldn't smell the cleaning agents when they walked in the door, they wouldn't feel the house was clean. Inversely, many people will mistakenly think their house is clean and be delighted when they walk into a gas cloud that could defoliate the Amazon.

That was then. Now after 20 years of eliminating poisons from use in my house, on my body, and in my food, I am shocked to discover how overpowering they are.

Just as people who live in towns with animal feed lots get used to the overwhelming and revolting smell of extraordinary amounts of fecal matter in the air, people get used to anything to which they're repeatedly exposed. (If you're unfamiliar with this smell, drive the I-5 between LA and San Francisco, and you'll pass a few of those towns—the memory will stay with you and make you reconsider your diet.)

Back to poisonous agents in our homes. Worse than smelling horrible and negatively affecting the health of the individual and the planet—they're unnecessary and waste our money! *How many reasons do we need to git it gone?*

As with most of my work, I like to rely on common sense, looking to nature for answers, and do my own studies to determine what's beneficial and what's harmful. With so many "studies" and "reports" sponsored by the very companies making the products being tested, self-reliance and smarts are a must.

With that in mind, I'll list some of the items that I've completely eliminated from my home. If you enjoy using these products, as I used to, consider giving them up (or just one of them) for a few weeks or months—just as a test to see if that Allie Chee is takin' this health thing too far or if she's on to something!

I thought it would be good to rank them in order of least necessary but couldn't decide which were least toxic and wasteful, so this is a list off the top of my head:

Dryer Sheets

I think these came to mind first because I smell them in the air every day when I stroll with my baby. Yes, in the air. I don't need to stand next to the dryer in the laundry room or even in the house... if someone has them in the dryer as I walk by their house, I smell them. As with other cleaning agents, I used to enjoy that "freshly washed smell" they imparted.

Now I feel sorry for people who pass me on the street, giving off particles of poisons to passers-by from their clothing and stinking up the environment.

Scouring Powders

We just talked about these, but unlike dryer sheets that serve no real use, these actually do something. If you have nasty gunk on your stove, bathtub, or toilet, they do help remove it. And so does good ole baking soda! You can put baking soda in your bread or muffins and eat it. But Ajax muffins or Comet scones?

Carpet Powder / Freshener

If there were ever anything invented nastier than this, I have yet to find it. Carpets alone are a highly questionable invention—made of toxic synthetic materials, flammable, and incredibly dirty no matter how often you vacuum. I'm baffled how we Americans can walk through every kind of schmutz in the subway and then go home and wipe those same shoes across our carpet and furniture.

And it gets worse. We move into homes with old carpet where countless people rubbed their shoe bottoms—oh, my! True, they've been "cleaned"—water and soap squirted on them and then suctioned out—but not completely. If you want to see a living, growing science experiment, look at a fiber of the padding under the carpet through a microscope.

There are countries that call us barbaric. When considering our carpets, they just might have a point. My cousin used to call carpet "the dirty socks you can never take off."

And to make it smell "fresh," people sprinkle (or douse) a powder of unknown chemical origin on top of the funk.

Putting in that tile floor is sounding better and better.

If we have carpets, the way to keep them clean—and from stinking—is to take off our shoes before walking on them and avoid spilling things on them. When I live in a dwelling that I'm renting and have no choice about the flooring, I lay rugs on the carpet—they can be removed, beaten outside, aired-out in the sun, and really cleaned.

Air Freshener

More ludicrous than carpet freshener is AIR freshener. Even if it's not fresh, what is fresher than air? Well, if the air in our homes isn't fresh, adding poison to the mix isn't going to help.

In Germany, I was amazed to find people walking through their homes every day upon waking and opening every single window—even in winter. This means that for months and months when it's 10-30 degrees, they open their windows and allow that crisp, truly fresh air to fill their home.

Where I was from, that could get you in trouble. Growing up in Texas, the refrain was, "Close that door quickly behind you—you tryin' to cool the whole neighborhood?" Homes were virtually sealed up year-round. Ditto for office buildings.

When I lived in Chicago, I worked in a building in which all the windows had been painted shut to "seal" them. Granted, it gets wickedly cold there, but air is air... and I want fresh air, scalding, freezing, whatever. I used a hammer and a screw driver to pry open all the windows in my office, and I might have been the only person in the city who did.

Somewhere along the way, some humans decided it was acceptable to live sealed up in boxes. Then, when those boxes started to stink, they started spraying chemicals to give them a "fresh meadow" smell, if only for a few minutes. Talk about an aberration.

Let's think outside the box—literally.

If it's the romance and sensual feeling of a pleasing smell we're after, I'd suggest burning essential oils or, in the case of incense, I know of one man who makes a product I'll put into the air in my house:

Fred Soll is a guy who lives in New Mexico. I've never met or spoken with him, but I've used his products, looked at his website, and spoken with his assistant—and he gets the "thumbs-up" from me!

The name of his incense? "Fred Soll's." He uses only natural resins, essential oils, and herbs. He hand rolls the incense sticks, dries them in the New Mexico sun—and they are a delight. He runs his company with the help of his wife, sister-in-law, and one part-time employee.

One time when I called to order, I said to his assistant, "I've had my favorites that I've burned for a long time. I want to try something new. What's Fred's favorite?"

She said, "Well, I don't know his favorite, but I do know that when he lights a stick of his Nag Champa lavender, he says to me, "We're gonna burn a little piece of heaven.""

Now when I light it, I turn to whomever is in my house, smile, and say, "We're gonna burn a little piece of heaven." In one minute, it imparts a rich, exotic feel to the house for the day. It's one of the tiny, simple, and almost-free ways I make my time in my house a sacred experience.

When the "smells" we add to our body and home are from natural sources, we are participating in an ancient and wonderful tradition—and a technique for healing and balancing—called *aromatherapy.* Anything else—*git it gone!*

Sunscreen

Here's a hot topic! If we have no choice whatsoever, then—and only maybe then—it may be a good idea to use this toxin that is now made with nanotechnology so we have zero clue how it will affect us or the environment. There are almost always options that allow us to avoid these nasty chemicals that harm not only us individually, but all life as well, starting in the waters where we wear them.

In Malaysia (my husband's birthplace), locals joke about the "lobsters" baking in the sun, meaning the tourists—mainly Caucasians from Australia, Europe, and the U.S. They have an expression about the sun burning (a.k.a., sun tanning) habits of the tourists: *Only mad dogs and Englishmen.* Meaning, only mad dogs and the English lounge in the noonday sun—the time when the sun's rays can be harmful, rather than beneficial, as they are at sunrise and sunset. The locals, with skin much more suited to exposure in the tropics, wouldn't think of lying in the sun at noon.

So how to avoid sunburn without sunscreen?

- Don't lounge in the sun at peak hours or for more than 15-20 minutes.

- Sit in the shade. (You still get some exposure in the shade so this must be done with caution at peak times.)

- Wear light clothing that covers the skin, including a hat. (I carry an umbrella, too, and everyone but the Chinese and a few Latinos laughs. No mind. I like using my "sunbrella.")

Doesn't that sound better than mysterious chemicals of questionable efficacy that harm us and wildlife alike?

Antiperspirants

This one's a tough sell. Just as we don't enjoy stinky carpets and air, we don't like *our bodies* to be stinky! There are also answers for this desire to smell fresh that don't require us to give ourselves breast or lymphatic cancer.

The body is meant to perspire and it should. We can allow it to and still minimize any unpleasant odor with these ideas:

- Use a deodorant-only product, avoiding antiperspirant.

- Better, use one of the products, like a salt crystal, that don't have long lists of chemicals.

- Best, if we're clean inside, we smell better outside. Granted, none of the body's waste and cleansing by-products— including sweat—smell like roses, but if we're eating well, exercising, and our hormones are balanced, our odors won't send everyone running for cover. Skipping deodorants and antiperspirants entirely, living healthily, and using a dash of natural essential oils makes us not only stink-free… there are many who would say the body's natural smell, with a dash of rose, neroli, or sandalwood is quite the turn-on— and I'm one of them!

Give it a try: let go of one toxic addition for just a week. See how sweet (smelling) life can be, *naturally!*

Our Home, Our Sanctuary

A friend from Israel told me, "I'm not getting married until I can be with a woman and know that 20 years later, just thinking about going home to her is going to make me push harder on the gas pedal."

Do we all risk traffic school to race home from work to see our families? Hopefully not, but do we *want* to race home? Does our heart beat faster just thinking about walking in the door? Or inversely but equally nice, does a warm calm come over us as we imagine a gentle evening with our loved ones?

It won't feel that way every day, but it can feel like that more days than it probably does now.

To repeat the point: We should feel at least the same amount of love and reverence when walking in our front door as we would walking into our church, temple, mosque, yoga school, and gym. Wouldn't it be great if we felt excited, inspired, and happy just thinking about being at home?

If so, then we need to approach the care, design, and

respect of our home sanctuary as we would a holy place, and let's start with…

- Do we see mega-wide screens blaring commercials for cleaning products and pharmaceuticals 24/7 in all the rooms of our temples?

- Do we leave dirty socks and underwear on the altar at church for the preacher to pick up?

- Are there weeds covering the front entrance to the meditation center?

There are lots of ways we can design, clean, furnish, and care for our homes that will impart a magical, reverent feel—and they'll be different for everyone.

A way to start working with this principle is to begin with one space. It could be the study, or the guest room could be converted to an art room or meditation room. Or it could even be a small section of the yard that you tend with care, planting your favorite flowers—the place you sit and drink tea in the morning.

One time I lived in a tiny apartment where the only space to spare was *behind* my bedroom door when it was shut. In that little nook of empty space, I made a special place where I would sit and read, chill, or pray. I propped a beautiful pillow against the baseboard, hung a gorgeous textile from Indonesia on the wall, I burned some of Fred Soll's incense, *et voilà*—my sacred space.

Look around your house, pick a spot, and ask yourself—does this look like a place that is respected as a place of worship? A sacred place? (Is that you giggling I hear?)

Then, go about making it sacred!

This is an activity that can't be measured by Western science, and there are no PowerPoints to prove its validity.

But there is a fascinating art practiced worldwide called Feng Shui. It's the ancient Chinese system of geomancy based on the laws of "heaven and earth" to create balance, peace, and positive energy flow in our environment (internal and external).

With or without a system, we can all feel the truth of the benefits for mind and body when creating sacred space and moments.

We can feel the love!

Our Daily Vacation in Beddy-bye Land

Some people rarely remember dreams, some remember them all the time, and some learn to be lucid participants and conductors of their dreamscapes. Utterly fascinating. I could read a book a month on sleep and dreams without tiring of the subject—it's one of our greatest mysteries.

I consider sleep the most incredible journey we ever take. After traveling for 20 years in wild and wonderful places, I still find dreamland the most mystifying, scary, beautiful, and enlightening place to go.

And we get to go, every night—*for free.*

Scientists will tell us we go there to heal, recharge, unwind the mind and body, and get ready for the new day. Mystics, yogis, and spiritual leaders tell us that we go there to learn about the multiple realms of "reality," to reach our infinite self, and to learn to die.

For whatever purpose we do go there, we spend one-third of our lives sleeping, so let's make the most of it for ourselves—and one another.

How do you prepare for bed? How do your family members prepare?

Many people end the day as unceremoniously as they begin it. Throw back dinner, maybe a quick shower, turn on the bedroom TV, flop in bed, roll over, toot (!), snore.

That's not a proper "bon voyage" for the evening journey. Shoot, even a dog stretches and fluffs his blanket a bit before drifting off.

Master Hua Ching Ni, in one of his many lectures on Taoist philosophy, likens sleep to a journey. He says that as with any journey, the better we prepare, the smoother the journey goes. With that in mind, make a checklist of things you will do before bedtime, just as you would to prepare for a trip.

My list includes some ideas from Western schools of thought, some from Eastern schools of thought—and some from just fun schools of thought—to make the last few minutes we share together each day more enjoyable, healthy, and even sacred.

- The last 30 minutes before bedtime: no viewing of screens which stimulate, making it harder to fall asleep, no discussion of anything negative or violent, and no rushing. Begin to wind down with soothing music, perhaps a warm bath, and reading from a book you find sacred or inspiring.

- Use pleasing fragrances to set the mood for peaceful sleep. Pick an essential oil that is soothing for you and use it in a lotion or oil to rub on your skin. Burn a candle and sit in quiet meditation. Spritz your sheets with an essential oil spray like lavender, vanilla, sweet orange, or neroli (bitter orange). Don't worry so much about what the fragrance is "supposed" to do—they're categorized by their calming or energizing effects—just use something that pleases and calms you.

- Back to grooming. Groom your family members. Brush each other's hair before bed. Give each other five-minute foot rubs. Hug and snuggle with each other; and tuck the kiddos in bed.

- Say prayers of gratitude in silence or out loud together. Review the day's bounty and give thanks. Feel joy and gratitude in every cell of your body like a glowing light. Wow, you'll be surprised how calming and relaxing that is. I'm typing right now in the shade of a palm tree while my baby naps in her stroller. Just thinking about *thinking about* gratitude, I feel like curling up with her and taking a blissful nap, too!

• Here's a technique I learned from *The Tibetan Yogas of Dream and Sleep* by Tenzin Wangyal Rinpoche. As you're lying in bed preparing for sleep, you may need to use a little discipline and technique to redirect your mind away from the grasping and aversion it carries from events of the day or in anticipation for tomorrow—the stuff that robs us of sleep or disturbs the sleep we do get. If you find any thoughts of grasping (anything involving a sentence that starts with "I want," "I need," or "I have to" are examples) or aversion (anything starting with "I hope he doesn't," "What if she," and "I'm in trouble if") going through your mind, set up your fortress of protection.

Your huh?

That's right—your own fortress of protection, guaranteeing your safe departure, happy travels, and peace and joy upon returning from dreamland.

If you're Catholic, you might visualize a circle of your favorite saints watching over you, your loved ones, and your house.

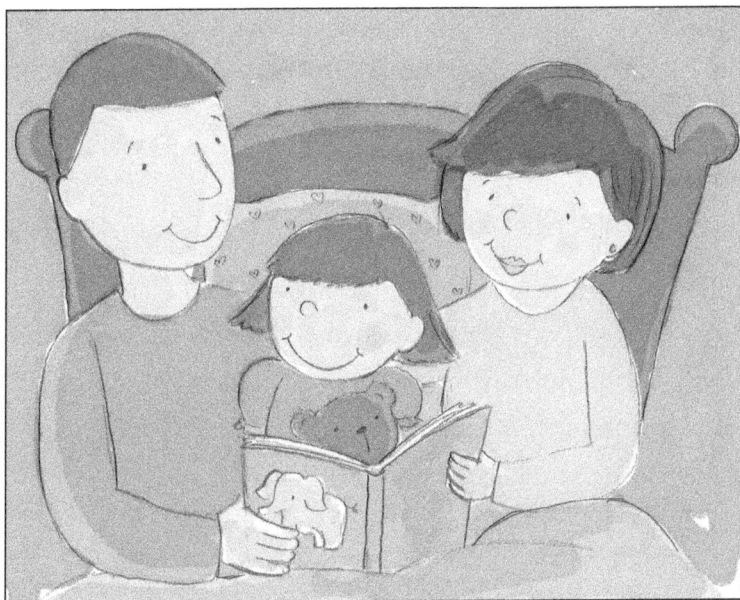

Loving bedtime rituals are the perfect way to end the day. It won't be just the children who look forward to them.

If you're Protestant, you might feel the presence of Jesus with you.

If you're Buddhist, a circle of Buddhas, Bodhisattvas, and Dakinis.

Other possibilities are an angel as a representative of Mother Earth watching over you, a Council of Wise Elders or your ancestors encircling you, or simply a sphere of impenetrable armor of white light emanating from you.

If you enjoy this technique, it's a great one to teach children—it can be especially helpful for them if they awaken startled from a dream or are scared of the dark.

And speaking of children...

I've always felt a little twinge of sadness when I witness parents shouting from the next room to their kids, "Time for bed. Lights out." Not even a kiss on the cheek? Not even a tuck of the blanket? No hug...? *No fun! No love!*

Until he was about nine, my nephew and I had one of the most elaborate bedtime rituals I've ever conjured up—we both looked forward to it every night.

It started with lighting the magic ocean candle. Then we'd discuss how people thought those things on their ceilings were lights and fans, but they were really travel machines, waiting to take us to Dreamland once we fell asleep. We'd discuss where we were going, if we'd meet there, or had different plans. (While he usually wanted to go to Candyland, I encouraged him to meet me in Veggieland.)

I'd spritz his pillows and bedding with sweet orange and vanilla aromatherapy spray to guarantee happy travels.

We'd hug, I'd tuck him in safely, making sure every toe was under the special organic Star Wars sheets I bought for him... *and then* it was lights out. That was fun, and not just for him!

Pick even one or two special things to do together at bedtime—and make it a routine for even one week. See if you don't find yourself feeling much more peaceful as your head hits the pillow, if your dreams aren't sweeter, and if you don't wake up feeling more refreshed.

We spend one-third of our lives in Beddy-bye land—just a little loving intention with that time can change the course of our lives.

You can keep it simple. Have a good pillow fight and pile on the *love!*

AROUND THE WAY

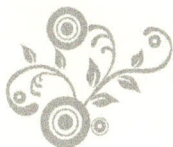

S imple and delightful ideas that anyone can implement—right now—to make their home and extended environment:

- *More supportive*

- *Happy*

- *And overflowing with love*

Mexico was the first country I visited outside the U.S. I was 19 years old and dating the son of an immensely wealthy man. Their family home was a sprawling estate in one of the best neighborhoods of Mexico City, Lomas de Chapultepec.

As is often the case with the generation that enjoys opulent wealth (as opposed to the generation that created it), he was an entitled shite and fancied himself a major "playa." However, I was (and remain) grateful for the experience of knowing him. I fell deeply in love—*not with El Cabron*—but with Mexico and a way of life entirely new to me.

His family gathered for breakfast, every day. A sprawling, fresh, intoxicating spread complemented with fresh juices of mango, coconut, guava, and papaya.

His family gathered at home again for lunch and again for dinner.

During these meals, they laughed, they talked about their day, they joked, and they spoke of politics, art, business, literature, and travel—in multiple languages.

Enchanting!

The family life, the focus on beautiful family meals together, the incredible depth of their education and culture—I was dumbfounded, especially since the perception I'd gained of Mexicans from the talk of the Caucasian population in Texas didn't include this particular rendition. Of course, I gained a skewed vision of the opulence with which the citizens of Mexico live, but the focus on family and meals together ran through the economic spectrum there, I later discovered.

I was not only dumbfounded... I felt a little... dumb. I didn't lack ability or willingness to learn—I'd just never been exposed to a people so multifaceted and fascinating. One evening at their ranch (one of the many estates they owned), as servants brought in a lamb that had been wrapped in banana leaves and baked in the Earth for 24 hours, one of the people in attendance suggested that everyone recite their favorite poem. And out came the verses in English, in Spanish, in French.

When the circle made its way to me, I thought of two lines from Ovid, a phrase from Walt Whitman, the title of a piece from Khalil Gibran—and I froze. The only complete work I could think of was "God is great, God is good, let us thank Him for our food." And for cryin' out loud, the endings are spelled the same but don't even rhyme!

It's not that I hadn't read classical literature—I was majoring in literature because of my love for it. I simply (very simply) had never been in an environment where people valued great and terrifying poetry to memorize and recite over a dinner of lamb slaughtered by their servants, baked in the Earth, and served in banana leaves.

I remember thinking it was a little ironic that the people I knew in Dallas—although many were hardworking and intelligent, they were monolingual, living on take-out pizza, lacked family life, and had traveled as far and wide as Fort Worth and Las Vegas—would speak disparagingly about the people (they'd never met) in Mexico. More than once I was asked with a look of disdain, "You mean to tell me you're datin' a Mexcan?"

When close friends and family would ask, "What's it like there?" I'd sum it up with "Mexico is so… different!"

A few years later, during my travels in Europe, with each country I'd say, "Wow, France is so different!" "Italy is so different!" "Germany, Turkey, and Greece are so different!"

Finally, a little light went on in my head. Maybe it wasn't that all the rest of the countries in the world were so different. Maybe it was the US… the youngest and most industrialized and materialistic of countries, that was *so different*.

My subsequent travels around the world have proven this to be the case, at least for this point of discussion.

What I learned changed my life. I saw people in 50 countries rich and poor living close to their loved ones, supporting one another, and living what appeared to be—from top to bottom—healthier lives.[16] Not all of them, of course, and they have their own issues. But my proposal is: why don't we keep all the wonderful advantages we have in our rich, powerful nation and also learn to build, appreciate, and reap the rewards of life with tight-knit families, friendly neighbors, and town centers—a "village" life.

I live in Northern California where there are millions of successful, intelligent people. Silicon Valley attracts some of the leading minds in the world who create great wealth here and around the planet.

Yet consider these experiences:

When my husband and I first moved to the East Bay in what was considered a desirable family town with an excellent school district, we'd seen neither hide nor hair of a neighbor for about a month. Deciding that we should

---

16. Some would say fortunately—I would say *unfortunately*—that has been changing rapidly in the 20 years since I started traveling. "Poor" countries, meaning those without a TV in every room of the house and a warehouse-style grocery store on every corner, have increasingly bought the story that their lives are inferior and have been ferociously building fast-food joints and malls where there were once beaches, town centers, and historical landmarks.

make the first gesture, we went to a friend's farm, picked baskets of beautiful fresh apples and arranged them in little baskets with a "Hello Neighbor" card in each one.

We knocked on the first door. No answer, so we left the basket on the step.

The next door, the woman (mid-30s, well dressed, holding her baby, BMW SUV in the driveway, perfect lawn), snatched the basket, and said, "Well, I've gotta go now," and slammed the door. She never so much as said "hello" in passing after that. (To be fair, maybe her meds weren't quite right.)

The third, fourth, and fifth doors—no one home, and again we left the baskets on the door.

After one month, we bumped into the fifth neighbor in her driveway. She said, "Oh, you dropped off those apples. Thanks."

And that was it. Of course with exceptions, but I've had similar experiences in neighborhoods all across America, from Dallas to Chicago and from Naples, FL to LA. In general, Americans aren't "close" with their neighbors.

(If you're shaking your head, reading this and thinking, "That's not so"—never leave your neighborhood!)

Other stories may happen, but *that kind of story* would absolutely never happen in almost any other country I've visited or lived in. In North Africa, the Middle East, almost all of Asia, and other regions of the world, it would not only be shameful to fail to greet new neighbors, but also impossible that a kind gesture from someone new would go unreturned or unacknowledged— *even if the locals had decided for any reason that they didn't like the new neighbors.*

Another story from my childhood.

I was a spindly kid and my best friend in grade school, as it turned out, was the heaviest girl in my class. We made quite a pair.

She and I were inseparable. When she found out I had to wait at the empty school grounds until my mother came to pick me up at 5:00 or 6:00 every evening, she got permission from her parents for me to go home with her after school and have my mother pick me up there.

We would walk or take the bus to her house, we'd eat a snack when we got there, then settle down to do our homework or go in the backyard and jump on the trampoline.

Her parents were upper middle class, meaning: they had a large, beautiful house and nice cars, mom was a housewife, dad was the manager of a successful investment firm—all was well. They knew my story: dad AWOL, single mom working long hours, no other family members to speak of. My clothes alone would tell the story: we weren't *dirt* poor, but we weren't playing tennis on the weekends either.

One day when we got to her house, my friend told me as she reached in the refrigerator for a snack, "My mom said you can't eat our food anymore." And that was that. I'd sit, hungry, and watch her eat every day after school.

Well, hey, I grew up with Wild West prairie life where it was every man, woman, and child for themselves—so at the time, I just felt ashamed—as if I'd done something wrong.

In hindsight, with more life experience, including being a mother, adoring children, and adoring cooking for children, I look at it from a slightly different angle.

The poorest people in the world wouldn't disgrace themselves by denying a visiting child a piece of fruit while their own child ate, even if it were every day. My travels proved that time and time again. The poorest of people will offer their best food, clothing, and shelter to visitors—even if the visitors are wealthy.

My husband, Malaysian, said any mother of his childhood, knowing that hungry children were on their way to her house from school would be busy in the kitchen cooking for them.

So why did I share that story in particular? There are many people who extend small gestures of kindness every day in many ways, but there are also plenty of folks who would think, "Well, hold on now… if that kid were there five days a week, I can see the parents not wanting them in their fridge."

And I don't think it's pure greed. I believe we just haven't been taught in our society, we haven't seen, and therefore we don't know how to live in true hospitality and community.

And I shared this story to say…

In the richest country on Earth, a well-to-do family can't spare a 10¢ piece of fruit for their kid's friend?

We can do better than that!

Hospitality.

Generosity.

Compassion.

Kindness.

The stuff of village life and the things that bring grace, honor, and joy to our daily lives.

I've shared a few stories of inhospitable behavior, so here are just a few stories of the thousands I experienced around the world, of gracious, effusive hospitality—of people who cherish community, family, and friendship. People who consider it a reflection of their personal honor and that of their family to be generous, helpful, and kind.

On my very first flight across the Atlantic, I sat alone among a group of French people who'd all been on holiday together in Mexico. They were sunburned, mildly intoxicated, playing cards, and passing food (I saw the contents of one basket that included a meat, a jar of mustard, a baguette, and a sprig of rosemary... *Oh-la-la!*) down the aisles and over chair tops.

That alone had me amazed. I'd only been off the ground 30 minutes and I was already in a different world.

When we landed, a young man and his mother—fellow travelers on that flight—saw that I was looking dazed about where to go for baggage claim. They approached, offered help, and started polite conversation.

The mother was wearing a stunning skirt suit and a *hijab* (the traditional Muslim headscarf—but I didn't know that term at the time), her son was dressed elegantly, and though their English was flawless, there was a slight accent. They asked how often I came to Paris, and I told them this was my first time overseas.

They both showed excitement for my new adventure and concluded, "If this is your first hour in Paris, then you can't refuse to join us for tea in a café, and then we will see you to your lodgings!"

I was thrilled. Here again, only hours away from Texas and already another world. Over tea I discovered they were the wife and son of the ambassador from Kuwait to the U.S.

In September 2000 I flew from Los Angeles to Panama City. Following my rules of traveling alone safely, I'd arranged my flights so I would land in the early afternoon in Panama with enough time to look around town and find a place to stay. As luck would have it, my plan of "landing without reservations, but with enough time to find a place" backfired. Landing here was slightly less safe for a woman traveling alone than, say, Paris or London.

During the stopover in Miami, the connecting flight was delayed several hours due to storms. I've never had a flight through Miami not be delayed because of storms—it goes with the territory—but this one was more serious. The connection to Panama left three hours late, which was going to put me on the ground at 4:00 p.m., rather than 1:00 p.m. Well, that would still leave some sunlight and "safe" time to look for a hotel.

Once in the air, I could see the reason behind the delay. There were magnificent, terrifying clouds that plumed thousands of feet in the sky, each with rays of sunlight and bolts of lightning crashing through them. They piled on top of each other as they approached the coast, creating a huge wall that eventually spilled over the top and looked like a five-mile-long tsunami breaking over the land. I felt blessed to see such a sight but wondered if it wouldn't be better to be bunking down in a Miami hotel and ordering room service.

As we approached Panama, the captain came on the intercom and said that the storms over Panama City were *really bad*, and that we'd need to circle for an hour or two until they passed. After those two hours, he came back on and said that the storms hadn't passed, we were too low on fuel to continue circling, and we were headed to Colombia.

The small circle of people on the plane that I'd befriended and I all shouted, "Colombia! Hooray!" For me, one country is as good as another when I'm on an adventure.

However, when we landed in Barranquilla, the captain said, "They don't have an immigrations office at this airport, so we have to stay in the plane on the tarmac. They're going to refuel us. In a few hours, we'll be back in the air to Panama."

Colombia at sunset or early evening was an exciting prospect. Panama, in the middle of the night, was not.

I sat contemplating my options and only came up with two ideas: Sleep in the airport or gamble on finding a decent cab and ask to be taken to a safe hotel. I turned to the Panamanian woman sitting next to me, Moritza, and asked which she thought was safer.

Without hesitation she said, "Girl, no way you're staying alone in the airport or going in a cab at 2:00 a.m. You're staying with my family tonight."

I was moved by her kindness and relieved, but slightly apprehensive when I saw her two 6'5" brothers pick us up at the airport. Even more so when I saw that their house, in the jungle, was literally wrapped in burglar bars. I decided no harm in asking, and Moritza explained, "The neighbors are nice, but we're close to the border with Colombia, you know." Now I knew.

At home, her mother tucked me in bed in my own room, (which I later found out was her bedroom—the nicest in the house), and I fell asleep to the sound of a million jungle animals and insects. In the morning, I awoke to a glorious sight: a sunny mist hung over their coconut, pistachio, mango, and banana trees.

Moritza's mother, all spunky 85 pounds of her, opened the door to my room, and salsa music blasted in from the kitchen where she'd been preparing breakfast for everyone. Wearing a nightgown and curlers in her hair, holding out a cup to me, she smiled and said: "Good mornin', child! You must be needin' the coffee after such a night!"

At breakfast, the family and I feasted on jungle fruits and Caribbean delights, we laughed, and they teased me for being "foolish" coming all the way to Panama without my family—it was like a gathering of long-lost friends.

As I turned to leave, I asked Moritza again, "Are you sure there's nothing I can do to show my appreciation?

Can I invite your family to dinner in town tonight? Breakfast tomorrow?"

She slapped my shoulder and said, "Girl, please. We are Panamanians. No problem."

I've lived that story, in some fashion, all over the world.

In this section, titled "Around the Way" (meaning anywhere we go once we've crossed the threshold of our front door), I share those ideas and ways of living that I've learned in my travels. I believe they create a more welcoming, supportive, loving community that can help us feel happier, safer, and healthier, around the way.

Make Just a Little Extra

In 2000, I lived in a stunningly beautiful 1890's historical building in Southern Cal in the San Gabriel Valley. It still had a hand-operated elevator and full-time elevator staff—in regal uniforms—to run it.

One of the gentlemen who worked the elevator was Thomas. He was in his mid-to-late 60's, highly dignified and well spoken, and always wearing a smile. He was single, worked the night shifts, and I knew he went home alone in the late evenings to an empty apartment. That's not to imply that he was lonely, but still... I've been single and eaten many meals alone. It gets old. If it goes on too long, it gets worse.

One night I tried a new dish and discovered that I'd cooked enough to feed myself, a few friends, and then

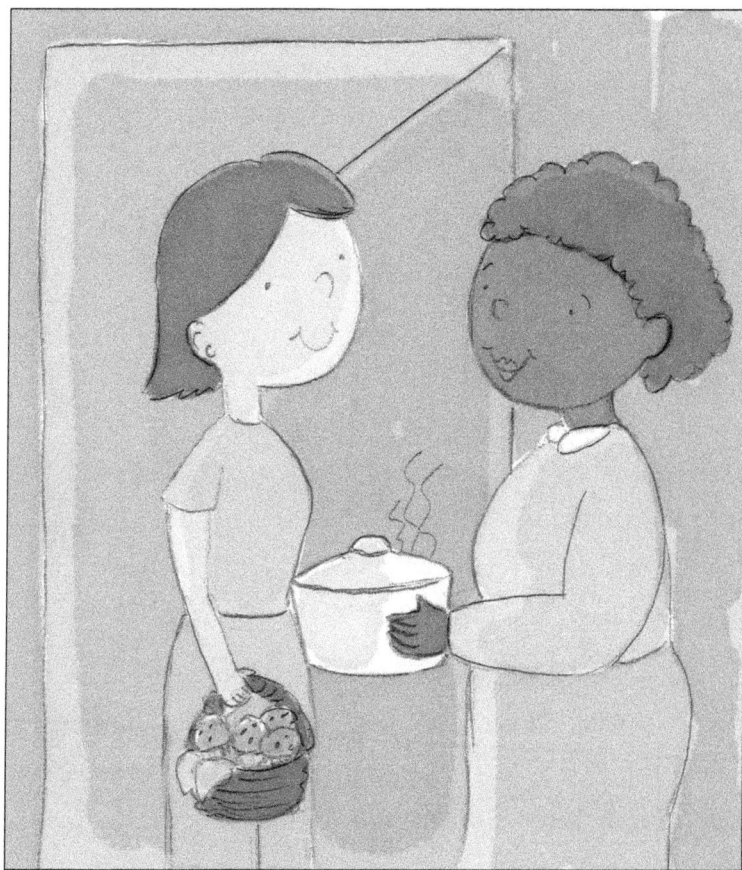

Small gestures of kindness and generosity go a long way in creating community.

some. Rather than stuffing it in Tupperware and forgetting it in the back of the fridge, I decided to put a serving in a lovely china bowl and deliver it to Thomas.

He accepted graciously with genuine gratitude. Doing that made me feel so happy that I began to make "special deliveries" to him several times a week. Sometimes a meal, sometimes just a cookie or piece of fruit. I don't know who was happier with the arrangement, him or me.

What I do know is that it was the beginning of a routine, so that now I regularly knock on neighbors' doors offering a bowl of soup, send my husband to work with some baked goodies for all his colleagues (that's made him popular around the office), or show up at friends' houses with a dozen eggs I hand gathered at the farm where I buy them.

I love it. Friends, neighbors, and family members love it. And even more fun… they begin to reciprocate. If you think your cooking is so-so, that magic ingredient "love" makes it taste a lot better to those eating it, and you'll bask in the joy you feel sharing it.

It's small. But it's a step in what leads to the healing and rebuilding of a village.

Who would've guessed? **Free love** *even in an elevator!*

On Holidays, Make at Least Five Calls

For most of my single life I was very happy to be single. But even being happy being single doesn't mean we don't get lonely—especially on holidays.

One of the worst holidays for me as a single person was Thanksgiving. It's not a romantic or festive holiday... it's a quiet, family holiday. If you have no family, it's a bummer holiday!

I'd always known, in some chamber of my mind, that I had thousands of reasons to be grateful every minute—thank you for my eyes that see the flowers, my ears that hear the birds, my nose that smells the ocean air—I had a long list, and I meant every bit of it. But one Thanksgiving morning in particular, in my heart I was lonely as hell and couldn't shake the feeling of *ingratitude.*

Then, as often happens in those moments, I thought back on my conversation with Mother Teresa.

Learn to love yourself, your family, your neighbors.

An idea popped in my head.

I had plenty of friends around the world who were single and without huge families—I would call everyone I could think of in that category and wish them a sunny, happy Thanksgiving.

With the first call, my mood lightened. With my second call, I felt "almost good." By the fifth call, I was positively elated and knew this would be a new tradition for me.

Remembering who might have just ended a relationship around Valentine's Day, remembering who's lost their father on Father's Day, remembering who's had a miscarriage on Mother's Day, and calling them to share love—it's a small way to make this a better world.

You Don't Have to Be *Like* Your Neighbors to Like Your Neighbors

If we rewind the clocks to the 1950's, we all, more or less, looked like our neighbors. If we didn't look exactly like them, we'd likely grown up in somewhat similar conditions with similar traditions. Even if we were Irish Catholics, the neighbor to the left was Polish Jew, and the neighbor to the right was African-American Christian—we were at least familiar with those people, places, and practices. Further, we (meaning the majority of people at the time) probably lived in the city or state in which we'd grown up. Even if we moved, it wasn't frequently.

Today, Americans move back and forth across the country like going for groceries. No roots—no community. Further, we have entire populations of people from every country on Earth in all the major cities in the U.S. These people don't just look different, they have religions a lot of people in the U.S. have never heard of or don't understand. They eat food we can't pronounce or identify. They dress differently. And, often, they're working on their English skills.

As many people do, I love that! I like to move frequently and discover new places; and I married one of those immigrants from a far-flung corner of the Earth (we're all in one of those corners—it's a matter of perspective).

But we need to consider the ramifications of these changes: it means that in a lot of cases we're not like our neighbors. BUT, that doesn't mean we can't like them! So how do we get to know them and like them?

I remember when whole blocks of neighbors would get together and play cards. Bridge was the rage with the adults when I was a kid. The neighborhood would gather in someone's living room or backyard, set up folding card tables, bring their beverages, and sit down for an exciting evening of bridge, conversation, and laughs.

Why don't we do that again?

It's a beautiful way to build community. You don't have to make much conversation—the cards make it. You don't need to be like each other, you don't have to go anywhere, and you don't have to spend any money.

If playing cards isn't your thing, a similar activity will achieve the same end. Whenever I move into a new neighborhood, I initiate Sunday "Grill-n-Chill" afternoons. It's informal, everyone has a standing invite, I supply the grill, one dish, and great music.

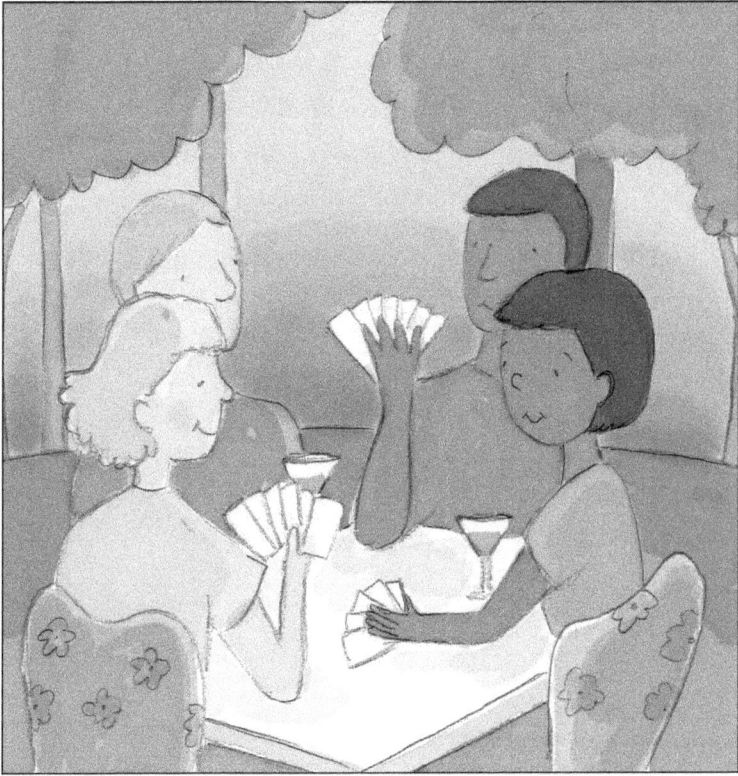

We don't even need to know what to say—we can let the cards do the talking!

People come and go during a set timeframe as they please. They can bring food to grill, they can bring as many people as they'd like, they can bring their kids and their pets!

It requires some effort to build momentum and attendance, but it's always worth it.

The mix of people and personalities at these gatherings is always different and always a blast. We never know where the conversation will lead or what connections and friendships will develop. I remember one of our best Grill-n-Chills was the day that someone brought bubbles (for one of the babies) and my dog entertained everyone by chasing and biting the bubbles as long as someone was willing to blow them.

Simple. Sweet. Love.

The Neighborhood Lawn Boy, Car Washer, and Pool Boy

If you're 35 or older and grew up in the suburbs (or at least in a neighborhood with lawns and pools), you'll remember that almost every street had "the guy"—or with me, the gal—who mowed neighbors' lawns, washed cars, or cleaned pools. It was usually the teenage son of one of the families on the street. Everyone knew him, trusted him, and was happy to help build his college fund in exchange for a mow, wash, or clean.

Where did these guys go?

My cousin used to be one of those lawn guys, and he built a successful business that put him through college. I asked him where those working neighborhood teens went, and here's what he said:

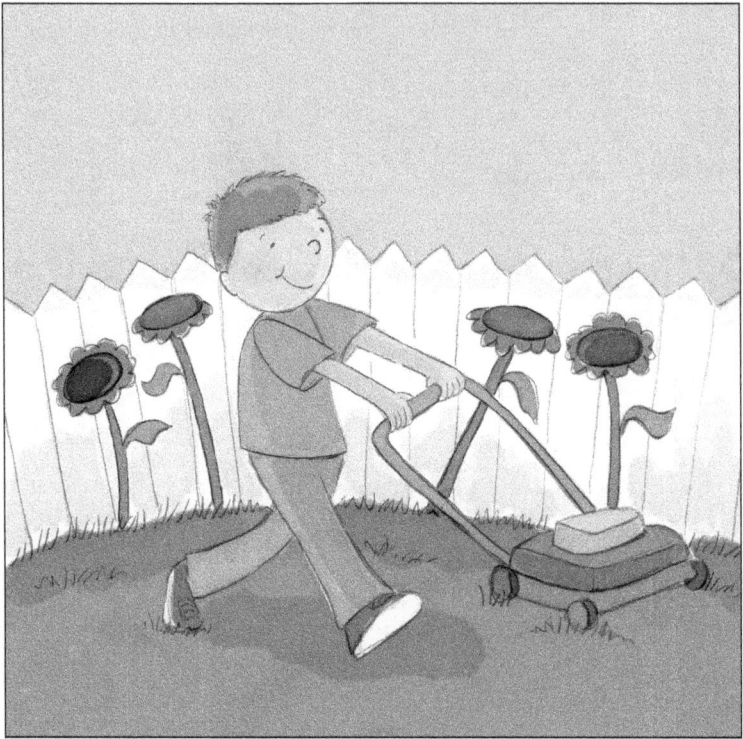

This used to be a common scene in the neighborhood—the neighbor's son mowing your lawn.

"There are two things that brought an end to the local biz for those neighborhood kids."

"The first was: parents stopped making their kids find jobs and earn money. I remember on the first day of summer vacation one year, my father kicked my brother and me out the front door at sunrise and said, 'Don't come back until you have jobs.' And we came back with jobs. That was when we were 14 and 16. Now, parents (except those who desperately need the money and often not even then) don't require their teenagers to get jobs on summer break, if ever. What are those kids doing now instead of working? My guess is: screwing around, getting in trouble, and losing themselves in online games and Facebook—it's what the guys mowing with me would have been doing if I hadn't given them a job. Of course, in our day it would have been Pac-Man."

"The second thing is that everyone became afraid of "liability issues" and lawsuits. Companies came in with teams of workers paid minimum wage. They had insurance and all the official papers, and somehow the whole country became 'afraid' to hire the teenage boy next door."

What he said rang of truth. "What does your teenager do during summer break and why doesn't he/she mow the lawn, clean the pool, and wash the cars for the neighbors?" I asked several parents around the country.

Here are just a few of the responses I heard when asking:

- *My teenagers spend the summer messing around with their friends.*

- *She goes to summer camp.* ["What do they do there?" I asked.] *They do... I don't know, lots of things. Swim, tennis, stuff like that.*

- *We have them do chores around the house, but we wouldn't want them bothering the neighbors about doing their lawns.*

- *He hangs out with his friends. He likes to sleep a lot during the day, but you know, he's a teenager.* [I don't know.]

- *I don't think it would be safe for him to walk around mowing other people's lawns.*

- *I don't really know what my kids do during the day—probably hang out with their friends, watch movies, read a little.* [Intrigued, I asked what they read.] *They're really into that teenage vampire genre.*

I'm not one of those people who likes to spread doom and gloom about the Asian Tiger children spending their time with their parents, ferociously learning advanced sciences and mathematics at midnight and on holidays, who will eventually take over America since we're all gluttons and lazy. But, hearing what I did from those intelligent, well-to-do American parents, I wondered if I should resume my private Chinese lessons.

When did it become acceptable to require *nothing* of young children and teenagers? Why are they considered lesser beings and incapable of accomplishment, drive, and contribution to the family?

I'm not a big flag waver, either, but just for this paragraph, I'm going to pull out the Stars and Stripes! America was founded and built into the greatest nation on Earth by people unafraid to break a sweat, with work ethics and commitment to growth and success (not all of them, but we're generalizing)… not by kids horsing around, getting fat, and reading (if) smutty vampire stories; and not by parents leaving the kids to do "whatever" with no guidance or requirements. The current generation of Americans is acting like the individual within a family that inherited wealth—and pisses it away.

It's not just the parents who've dropped the ball with their kids—it's the schools, too. PE class has been eliminated entirely or reduced to "hit your friend in the head with a ball" class. Ask any teenager you know to do 25 push-ups and sit-ups. If they can do it, it's probably not a result of training in PE class. Music class has nothing to do with learning to play an instrument or understanding music theory. It's "clap and sing" class. Then, with a recess period, a snack break, and a lunch break… there is a total of about one to two hours of real learning time in the school day.

We don't need to know higher mathematics to know the result of that equation over time.

Even if we don't want our children being officially employed while in school, and even if we don't want them to work around the neighborhood, we can at least require that they contribute to the upkeep of our—their own—dwellings.

- Have your son mow the lawn, wash the car, and sweep out the rain gutters.

- Have your daughter pick weeds, vacuum out the car, and sweep the garage.

I have interviewed dozens of women in the last two years to help in my home. Most were highly intelligent, but painfully ignorant. I wonder what skills they are going to bring to their lives as wives and mothers: "I can text faster than anyone I know and can rock a Facebook page like nobody's business! Wanna build a family together?"

I haven't interviewed young men to help in my home, but I'm sure the same applies to them as well.

The candidates haven't known how to separate clothes for laundry; or how to wash, chop, or cook veggies—one I hired cut off and threw away the tops of asparagus and kept the inedible base of the stems. She was a college senior in Silicon Valley and had never seen asparagus before. Or how to wash or assemble a blender, handle knives, or load a dishwasher. They certainly don't know how to check the chemical levels in a pool, start a lawn mower, or wash a car. I've had to teach my help—intelligent, college graduates—how to put soap in the dishwasher and *how to use a sponge*. They're being paid very well to receive training they should have had as children in their homes—and for which they should be paying me.

Learning these bare-essential skills not only helps support the family. It makes for a people—a nation—of self-respecting, capable, and responsible citizens.

Accomplishing that is a big leap toward restoring loving community.

Give It Away

Lots of folks donate time to charitable organizations, and lots of people write checks to their charities of choice. That is an important contribution to society and it's wonderful to support organizations working to make this a healthier, happier world.

In Laguna Beach, I met a man named Kip whose trademark was *extraordinary* generosity. I'm not talking about participating in charity bike rides and making donations—which he did all the time. I mean that almost every interaction with Kip left a person better off, financially, physically, emotionally, or all of the above!

I'd only heard about Kip from a friend, Steven. One day Steven took me to visit him, and when Kip opened his front door, Steven said,

"Oh man, that is an awesome leather jacket!" (It was very hot.)

Kip said, "You really like it?"

Steven said, "It's the coolest jacket I've ever seen."

Taking it off and handing it to Steven he said, "Then it's yours!" And he wouldn't allow Steven to decline.

Not something you see every day.

At the time I thought, "Wow, they must be best friends. He just gave Steven a jacket that cost at least $2,000.00." I also thought, "Maybe this guy's completely loaded and it just doesn't mean much to him."

Later I discovered that they were very good friends but that Kip would do similar things with total strangers. Further, I discovered that, yes, he was well-to-do, but that he was self-made and had come from a modest upbringing. What he had he'd earned with years of dedication to his work.

Kip and I became friends and as I spent more time with him, I saw many more acts of spiritual and financial generosity.

Any time he was invited to a person's home for dinner, he'd bring a basket—one of his trademarks was an enormous basket he'd filled with things he believed the recipient would enjoy. And not just fruit or wine. Expensive clothing, books (self-help and health topics), accessories for the home, even the latest electronics.

When he would meet a client, instead of going *for coffee*, he would invite them to meet *for shopping at a health food store!* They would always accept—curiously— and he'd cut business deals with the CEOs and directors of huge companies, while encouraging them about which supplements were ideal for their body type and admonishing them to eat more veggies while he bought organic produce for them!

Now you really don't see that everyday.

That's Kip.

It's not in all our natures to burst through doors carrying $1,000 baskets of high-fashion clothing and vitamins for our hosts and business partners—but what if we decided that we'd show up with a card written from the heart or a flower?

Love, love, and more love!

Really **Random Acts of Kindness**

I mentioned earlier that the word "kind" means "child" in German. Thus, we can look at "kindness" as "child-like."

I had a neighbor in LA from Iran named Sunny who was amazing in a hundred ways. She had the Midas touch in business, was an accomplished artist, a world traveler—and she had a wicked tongue, brilliant humor, and an ability to entertain that you rarely see other than in Ginger Rogers movies.

Despite all that, she was amazingly child-like... or kind.

She did the funniest things—things one would expect from a precocious, fun-loving kid.

One day while watering the plants on my balcony, I saw a strange life form emerging from the soil in which I had a small star pine growing. (Poorly, I might add. Trees want to be in the Earth, not pots.) It looked like a tuber or vine, but the skin was speckled like a leopard.

"What in the world?" I wondered.

Over the next few days, it grew several inches and a huge bulb, ready to burst, appeared on the end. It looked like an alien life form and I thought, "Maybe I should bring in a HAZMAT team or NASA." Its evolution became the major excitement of each morning.

At the end of about a week or so, I woke to a miracle. On my balcony, sitting next to my star pine in its big clay pot was the most stunning flower I'd ever seen. It leapt from the pot like a flame, and from the center emerged an enormous stamen that pointed toward the heavens. It was the richest burgundy color I'd seen in nature. I sat drinking my morning tea staring at it and wondering, "Where did you come from?" The color alone put me in a blissful mood.

Later that day Sunny popped by and I pulled her immediately to my balcony to see the vision. She laughed and said, "How delightful! Your voodoo lily bloomed."

"Voodoo lily? How do you know what it is?" I asked, not particularly surprised that she knew, since that was *so* *Sunny* to know.

She said, "Because, darling, I put it there."

She explained that since she was in her 20's (which I presumed meant around 30 years back, though I didn't know exactly), she would carry flower seeds and bulbs in her purse—even when traveling overseas. As she walked by a stray pot, window flower box, or bare patch of dirt, she'd reach in her purse, grab a seed or bulb, and drop it in. Then, a few days, weeks, or even months later, the owner of that pot or patch of dirt would find a colorful surprise.

To illustrate, she opened her fabulous designer purse to show me that she was carrying yellow tulip bulbs. She tossed a few on my coffee table and told me to give it a try.

She went on, "That reminds me, dear, I came over to tell you I'm going out of town and to ask you for any dresses or accessories that you don't use anymore."

As I started to dig in my closet, she explained why.

"When I have extra room in my suitcase, I always take dresses, scarves, and whatnot (her "whatnot" was everyone else's *haute couture*) when I travel to leave in the hotel rooms for the maids."

I'd heard my yoga teacher say during a lesson one day,

"Leave a wake of beauty behind you"

... and it stuck with me. It popped back in my head during this conversation with Sunny. She was quite literally leaving a wake of beauty behind her.

We don't need to leave flowers and high-fashion apparel for strangers to find and delight in—though it's a *super-sunny* idea! We can come up with our own signature random act of kindness.

Doing it will guarantee more smiles and love around the way.

End the Day with *La Passeggiata*

La passeggiata is the Italian social ritual—the art, actually—of taking an evening stroll.

Bellissima!

Living in Europe and traveling all over the Mediterranean, I refined my practice of *la passeggiata*. From Desenzano, Italy to Dalyan, Turkey to Beirut, Lebanon, to Sidi Bou Said, Tunisia—when the blazing sun goes down and the cool winds of sunset start to blow, *la passeggiata* begins. But the Italians have no rivals in the world for how beautifully they do it.

What does it look like? Babies, grandparents, teenagers hoping to score (at least looks) from the opposite sex, grandmas in way-high heels, old men wearing elegant hats, youths in the hottest fashion.

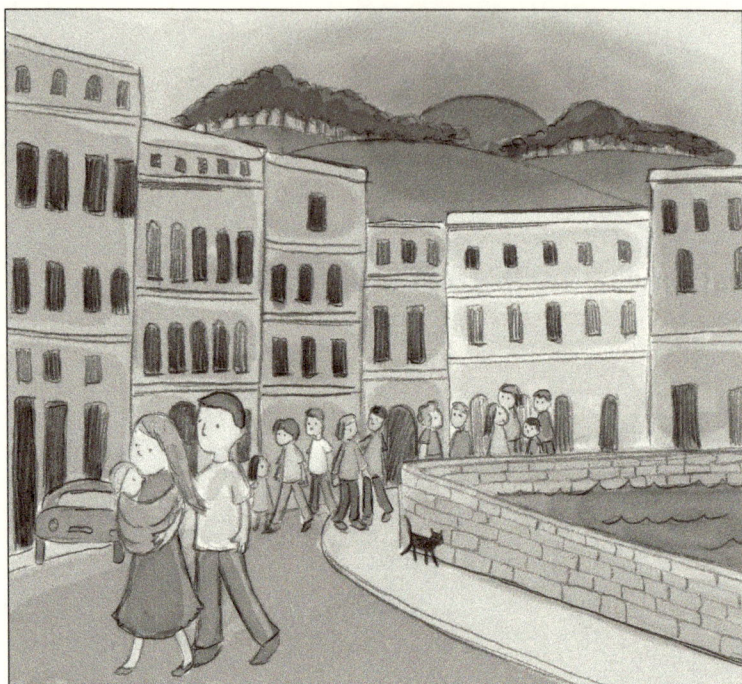

La Passeggiata... free love for all!

What are they doing? Strolling the piazza and the boardwalk, sitting at the fountains, eating gelato, gossiping, flirting, and enjoying their town and each other.

Before living in Italy, I'd already discovered the joy of an evening walk after dinner, around dusk, before bed.

In Long Beach, I was cycling through what we call one of those "down parts" of the up-and-downs of financial life: working long hours with no spare time or money for entertainment. But that doesn't mean I didn't have lots of love- and fun-filled days!

During this time I really turned up the volume on studying nutrition, using cookbooks, making wonderful new dishes every night, and then after dinner, strolling through the neighborhood and along the beach. I didn't have a fun name with lots of vowels for it, I just called it "going for a walk." And the beach part—that's so obviously beautiful— so let's talk about what I experienced and learned around the neighborhood.

I discovered the little details of my neighbors' homes: the architecture; the paint; the cleanliness or the sloth; changes they made to their gardens; and the way their gardens bloomed, died, and changed with the seasons.

Every house reflected the spirit of the people dwelling within. Over the months, those that were striking for one reason or another received nicknames: the "Free Tibet" house (a few flags), the "really Gay Pride" place (lots of flags), the haunted house, the house of a million roses, the place where the drummer for *Sublime* lived, the surfers' house, the cactus and succulent place, the cat house (*how many* cats lived there?), the "turtle mansion," and more. Even though I didn't know any of these people in the beginning, I began to feel a part of the community and to follow their lives.

When the surf was up, I knew I'd find dripping wetsuits hanging over the balcony at the surfers' house.

When fall arrived, I knew the elderly lady, who never came out of her hundred-year-old house into her tangle of thousands of ancient rose bushes, would finally emerge and do her annual pruning... before letting it go wild again for another year.

As I walked down the block, I knew from under which bush, at which house, which cat would emerge, to follow me— *only so far*—until we reached the point that was another cat's turf.

I lived two blocks inland, where the houses were beautiful 1920's Spanish style buildings—and affordable. As one walks the short two blocks toward the beach, the homes quickly become mansions. The walk from my place to the beach led by one beautiful and immaculately maintained mansion, with an exactly matching "itty-bitty" mansion in the backyard that was their pet turtle's house. One day, they had a sign posted on their beautiful wrought iron fence that said, "Reward for Information Regarding Our Family Turtle—He's Been with Us a Decade."

I mourned with them.

If I didn't see one of the cat "regulars" out for a nightly prowl for a while, I would wonder about them and feel joy when I would see them again.

I would share the owners' pride and happiness when they made significant and beautiful changes to their lawns and gardens.

I began to greet not only the people, but also the parrots, the palm trees, and the bougainvillea as dear friends.

I began to slowly feel not just a part of the neighborhood, but a part of *everything*.

And that takes us back to the beginning, to my hour with Mother Teresa, and to our collective life journey—which can be much sweeter, immersed in *free love at the hearth, at home, and around the way!*

The first light of dawn was filtering through the curtains. Without any thought, I felt, I knew, that there is infinitely more to light than we realize.

That soft luminosity filtering through the curtains was love itself.

— Eckhart Tolle

The Power of Now

GIVING BACK

A portion of the proceeds from *Free Love* is donated to **Growing Power.**

Growing Power transforms communities by supporting people from diverse backgrounds and the environments in which they live through the development of Community Food Systems. These systems provide high-quality, safe, healthy, affordable food for all residents in the community. Growing Power develops Community Food Centers, as a key component of Community Food Systems, through training, active demonstration, outreach, and technical assistance.

Will Allen, founder, farmer, and CEO believes, "If people can grow safe, healthy, affordable food, if they have access to land and clean water, this is transformative on every level in a community. I believe we cannot have healthy communities without a healthy food system."

Growing Power's goal is a simple one: to grow food, to grow minds, and to grow community.

For more information, visit **www.growingpower.org.**

CONNECT WITH ALLIE CHEE

Website

www.alliechee.com

Blog

www.freelovebook.blogspot.com

Facebook

www.facebook.com/FreeLoveBook

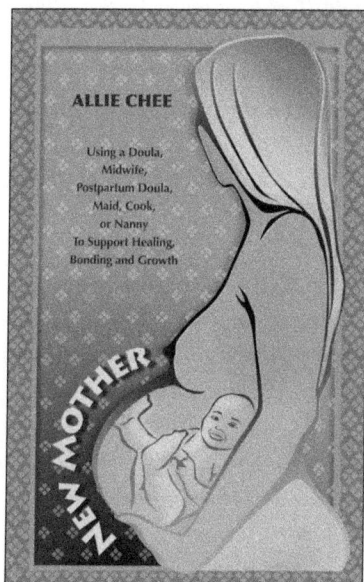